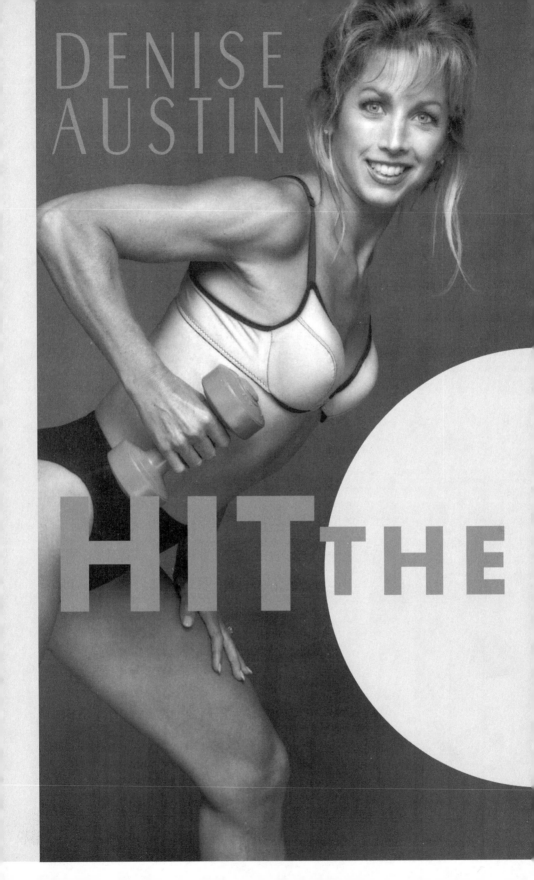

DENISE
AUSTIN

HIT THE

HOW TO TARGET,
TONE, AND SLIM YOUR
PROBLEM AREAS

SPOT!

A FIRESIDE BOOK

PUBLISHED BY SIMON & SCHUSTER

FIRESIDE

Rockefeller Center
1230 Avenue of the Americas
New York, NY 10020

FIRESIDE and colophon are registered trademarks
of Simon & Schuster Inc.

Designed by Barbara M. Bachman
Illustrations by Jackie Aher

Exercise photos throughout and frontispiece by Mary Noble Ours
Photo on page 12 by Charles Busch
Photo on page 18 by Timothy White
Other photos used by permission

Manufactured in the United States of America

1 3 5 7 9 10 8 6 4 2

LIBRARY OF CONGRESS
CATALOGING-IN-PUBLICATION DATA

Austin, Denise.
Hit the spot : how to target, tone, and slim your problem areas /
Denise Austin.
p.   cm.
1. Reducing exercises.   2. Exercise for women.   I. Title.
RA781.6.A89 1997
646.7'5—dc21   96–45162
                                                      CIP

ISBN 0-684-80218-X

To Jeff, Kelly and Katie

who

"Hit the Spot"

... the bottom of

my heart...every day!

ACKNOWLEDGMENTS

Always I think of my mom first when it comes to thanking people. She's been my true inspiration . . . she brought up all five of us kids by herself and did a great job . . . and thanks to my dad who taught me to always do my very best and that work can be a joy.

And a special thanks to my husband, Jeff, who honestly is the best! He is so supportive and wonderful. I am truly blessed to have him and our two girls, who light up our life. Thank you Jeff for everything.

To all my sisters who are always so proud of me. They are really my best friends! And to my brother who has so much patience with all of his four "loud" sisters.

A big thanks to Stephanie Mansfield, who helped me write "Hide the Spot," for her style, intelligence and expertise with the top magazines, including *Vogue* . . . she knows her clothes. I am fortunate to have Stephanie as one of my closest friends and godmother to my daughter Katie.

Thank you to Colleen Pierre, registered dietitian and spokesperson for the American Dietetic Association, for help in planning my "Hit the Spot" Pyramid Diet.

I would like to thank Sarah Pinckney, my editor at Simon & Schuster, for all of her help and support in this second book. And thanks to Jan Miller, my literary agent, who is my "head cheerleader."

There were so many days and nights that I spent working relentlessly on this book, so many times I would have rather been playing with my girls, or spending more time with my husband . . . but like so many working moms I have to juggle it all. I recall many a Saturday morning trying to write this book with my work spread out on the kitchen table, Katie sitting on top of my papers eating her pancakes, and Kelly tugging on my pajamas to get dressed and take her to the park. But even in the midst of this "juggling," every time I read a letter from a person who is looking and feeling better because of my TV show or my videos or books, it is a great feeling to know I have made a difference in her life . . . and that is what keeps me going and makes it all worthwhile.

How could a job be more gratifying . . . helping people feel better about themselves. I want to thank all the people who have written or stopped me wherever I am to tell me their success stories.

It is great to be appreciated . . . thanks!

CONTENTS

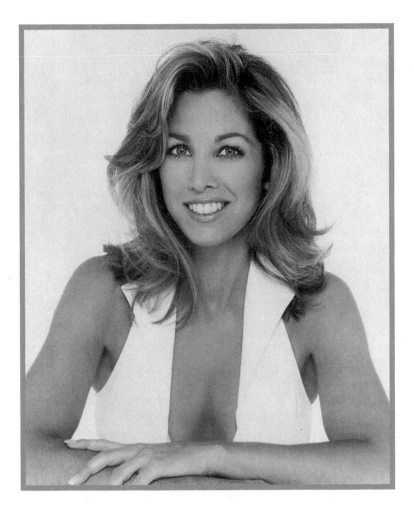

INTRODUCTION

There is not a woman on the face of the earth who is 100 percent satisfied with every inch of her body. If you asked any of your friends if they had a body part they would like to change, the answer would be "Yes!" Even supermodels complain about some part of their bodies.

Let's face it. *Nobody's* perfect.

Even I wish there were things I could change about my body. But imperfection is part of being human; the only way to be beautiful is to feel *good* about yourself and exude a positive outlook and a life-affirming energy for others. We are our own worst critics—no one else notices the flaws that we do. This can sometimes make us feel insecure about our bodies. Even the most beautiful woman feels vulnerable about certain things she would change.

How many times have you said, "If only I had a flatter tummy? . . . A smaller waistline? . . . Thinner thighs?" A tighter tummy will *not* make your life perfect. But it will make you feel stronger and more confident about your ability to change your life. This can help you alter your eating habits, your exercise schedule and your wardrobe choices.

Every woman has "a spot." There are many solutions to your spot problems, and this book maps out a step-by-step plan: Hit the Spot exercises, Hit the Spot diet and Hide the Spot tips on what to wear to flatter your figure. This three-part plan will target, tone and slim your problem areas. . . . we will solve them together!

And that doesn't mean spending hours every day in the gym. Let me be your personal trainer in the privacy of your own home. Share with me your problem areas and we will work together to tone, firm and reshape those spots.

Sagging arms? We'll firm them up. Drooping bottom? We'll lift it up. Flabby tummy? We'll tighten it up. Cellulite thighs? We'll smooth and tone them up. I will teach you to concentrate on the right spot.

We'll start with exercise. Even the busiest person can find time to "Hit the Spot." These are fast, effective shape-up ways to whittle your waistline, tighten your tush, resize your thighs. . . . all in just five to ten minutes a day. You'll learn exercises for your abs, your hips and thighs, buns, arms and bust!

What you put in your body is just as important as how you move it. You will love my easy eating plan, which allows you to create your own custom diet based on your weight-loss needs. I've created Crave Stoppers: chocolate, creamy, salty and crunchy treats that average only one hundred calories. These are already calculated into your daily healthy eating plan, which is based on the food pyramid, with a simple mix-and-match exchange program. Most diets fail because they are too stringent. My plan encourages you to eat well 80 percent of the time and to reward yourself with something yummy 20 percent of the time.

I know you will love my 7-Day Hit the Spot Eating Plan. These are my favorite recipes for delicious meals and snacks that my family adores. They will speed you on to a trimmer, healthier body.

One way to instantly slim your figure is to wear the right "Hide the Spot" clothes. So many women spend hours exercising and dieting and then choose an outfit that doesn't flatter. I want you to feel confident about your body, and to show off your figure! There is nothing more rewarding than finding an outfit that instantly makes you look five pounds slimmer. I will show you the fashion secrets, the "Do's and Don'ts" and tips to flatter any figure. There are ways to hide your flaws while calling attention to your best features. These are simple, fast, effective slimming tools every woman should learn. There are Mid-Section Miracles, ways to Disguise Your Thighs, and a new Rear View, all as a result of choosing the right clothes.

Although there is not a woman on earth who is 100 percent satisfied with her body, you will be 100 percent satisfied with my plan and you will see results in as quickly as 21 days.

Imagine—in only three weeks, you can have a sexier, firmer body! Yes, you *can* change your spots. And that's a perfect spot to be in!

Hit the Spot is working for thousands of people (you'll hear about their success stories in this book). They are losing weight, losing inches, and most of all, they are feeling better about themselves. Now you can do it too!

HERE'S HOW IT WORKS

Our muscles are what give our body shape. The only way you will ever improve and change your shape is by developing more muscle. Think of your muscles as modeling clay. You can form it, shape it and sculpt it the way you'd like. . . . It's the same with your muscles. It is all determined by the way you exercise. If you do not exercise, your muscles will become soft and flabby, but if you do specific exercises, you can shape, sculpt and form your body beautifully. Remember, you control the outward appearance of your body. The general features and inherent chemistry are genetic. You cannot change the framework—your bone structure—that you owe to your parents. However, you *can* change your muscles. You have over 640 muscles in your body, which you can reshape and tone, and as these muscles adapt to your new "Hit the Spot" exercises they will become strong and firm.

Muscle toning is the key to your fountain of youth. If you have firm, toned, tight muscles, nothing can droop or sag. Keeping your muscles firm will help prevent the pull of gravity. Strength training, resistance training, weight training, calisthenics—these Hit the Spot exercises are all muscle toning . . . and I'm not talking about body building or anything "macho" here; I just want you to tone up and firm up, to stay younger looking . . . as long as possible.

This book maps out a step-by-step plan—the Hit the Spot exercises, a Hit the Spot diet and Hide the Spot tips on what to wear to flatter your figure.

"MUSCLE TONING IS MY SECRET TO LOOKING YOUNGER"

D E N I S E   A U S T I N   (A G E   4 0)

MUSCLE TALK

Muscle cannot turn into fat and fat cannot turn into muscle. They are two entirely different tissues. When you do not exercise and have no muscle, you burn fewer calories and store more fat. When you gain muscle, your body burns calories at a faster rate. One of the main reasons we gain weight as we grow older is that we have lost good muscle tone. You can boost your metabolic rate just by adding more muscle to your body. So, get off that couch and develop those muscles. Fat cells are very sedentary where muscle cells are very active. . . . 24 hours a day. In turn, if you stop exercising, your muscles will shrink and you will probably gain fat. So, when you work on a certain part with the "Hit the Spot" exercise routines, you actually stimulate the muscles in that specific spot. First, you increase blood flow and circulation, and second, you command that specific muscle group to respond, firm and grow more muscle cells in your body. The more muscle you develop, the more calories you burn even while you sleep! Spot training really works! It changes undesirable spots into perfectly formed sexy spots.

MUSCLES WORK MIRACLES ON YOUR METABOLISM

The concept of working one specific body part has been around forever. All champion body builders work on one part at a time. Everyone who works out in a gym knows that working one body part at a time produces the most noticeable results in the shortest time period. Most exercise machines are especially designed to target and strengthen a specific body part or muscle group.

You can reshape and spot your body for a sleeker, sexier you! No matter how old you are or what type of physical condition you are in, this easy and very effective spot training can help you achieve dramatic results. . . . in just ten minutes a day. Stay young through "Hit the Spot."

WHAT ABOUT SPOT REDUCING?

I know you have heard that it's impossible to spot reduce. Well, this is true if you are just dieting alone and not exercising specific areas—dieting alone can only do so much. Of course, you will lose weight. However, without Hit the Spot exercises for those troublesome areas you cannot obtain the toned body that you want. You can not lose weight within one area of the body or lose fat in one area, but by following my exercise routine, you can have new tone underneath your fat layer. Your body fat percentage will decrease throughout your entire body.

There are three factors in getting rock-hard abs, perfect buns and thinner thighs . . . it's a 3-prong attack:

1. **Aerobic/cardio workouts at least 3 times a week for at least 20 minutes each time (see page 132 for aerobic options)**

2. **Good eating habits—follow my Hit the Spot pyramid diet (page 149) for healthy meals.**

3. **Hit the Spot: Muscle Toning exercises that zero in on your problem areas.**

It's a combination of all three . . . to get the perfect spot.

The Hit the Spot exercise section maps out a step-by-step plan of specific exercises for targeting those troublesome body parts: the abdominals, the hips and thighs, the buttocks and the arms and bust. Each exercise has simple, detailed instructions taking you through the entire movement, plus a picture illustrating the exact way I perform the exercise.

Once you have mastered the basic movement, try my variations listed with the exercise instructions. Each variation provides either a more intense version of the basic movement or a version that offers the use of a prop, such as a chair, to aid your movement.

This Hit the Spot section has my hand-selected favorite exercises . . . all to make you look and feel better. I would like you to try them all. Remember, concentrate on the muscles you are targeting. To make each body part look its best, make sure to vary your daily routine. Try not to get into a rut of doing the same toning exercises day after day! While each exercise and its variation do work one specific area, each variation is also unique in that it works the muscle in a slightly different manner, forcing it to adapt and become stronger, resulting in a more beautiful and sexier muscle. Also, changing your routine often keeps exercising fun and you motivated!

Pick and choose, mix and match—customize your own routine. I have even given you my personal ten-minute routine that I follow religiously. It is on pages 129-131, Sample Workouts. Even though week one, two and three are progressive, you can repeat the three weeks over and over again for variety and to hit those spots.

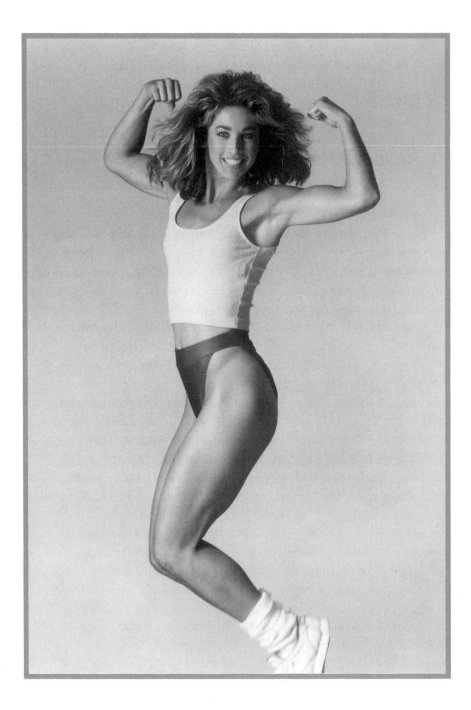

GET READY TO HIT THE SPOT

Here are five tips to get you started!

Make your mind up right now to start today . . . Only 10 minutes a day! You have 10 minutes to firm your thighs or arms or buns or abs. . . . It's worth it . . . because . . . you are worth it!

1. **Unplug your telephone so you won't be disturbed.**

2. **Find a spot in your house where you can spread your arms and lift your legs. It would be great to be in front of a mirror to check your form.**

3. **Wear a workout outfit. It gets you psyched up and puts you in the mood to exercise. Wear comfortable shoes (try my new Denise Austin cross trainers). Remember, the second you lace them up you are ready to go!**

4. **Try to do the 10-minute Hit the Spot routine at the same time each day so it becomes a habit, just like brushing your teeth.**

5. **You can do my Hit the Spot exercises any time of the day. You can even split it up: do 5 minutes in the morning to get you going or do 5 minutes in the afternoon when you feel a bit sluggish—it will rejuvenate you. Or do 5 minutes in the evening to release pent-up stress from work. Remember, even just one minute can help!**

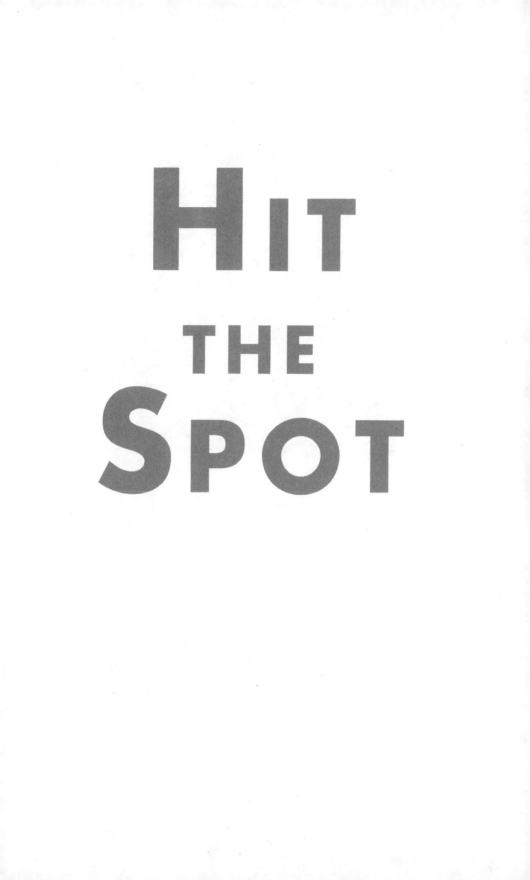

HIT
THE
SPOT

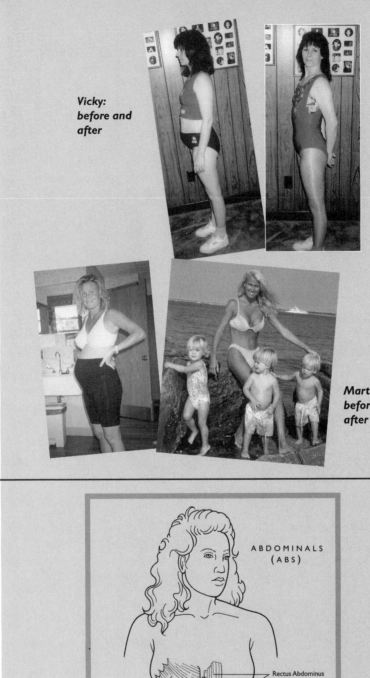

Vicky:
before and
after

Martha:
before and
after

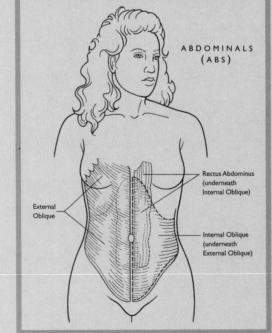

ABDOMINALS
(ABS)

Rectus Abdominus
(underneath
Internal Oblique)

External
Oblique

Internal Oblique
(underneath
External Oblique)

DEAR DENISE,

After having three children, two caesarean, I thought I would always have my big tummy. Not anymore! I do your Hit the Spot abs quite often and it works! I lost two inches from my stomach the first month. I enjoy watching and listening to you because you seem like a real person. You are interested in helping others become better people. Thank you for being an inspiration to myself and my children! I'll continue to exercise and be a better person.

JUDI—EDEN PRAIRIE, MINNESOTA

DEAR DENISE,

I love working out with you and Hit the Spot abs! After having triplets I knew I was going to have a tough time getting back into shape but with the help of your ab workouts I got back into my bathing suit in no time flat!

MARTHA—ALEXANDRIA, VIRGINIA

DEAR DENISE,

I am so happy I lost three inches of flab from my waist in just one month. Thank you Denise!

VICKIE—CINCINNATI, OHIO

For every inch your waistline exceeds the size of your chest, you can deduct two years from your life expectancy. Keep those abs fit—no other body part indicates a person's level of fitness as precisely as the centerpiece of the torso. . . . the abs!

Let's say goodbye to your paunch once and for all! Number one on everyone's wish list is to have a toned, tight, flat, sexy stomach! The good news is that the abdominal muscle is an area of the body that responds particularly well and quickly to exercise, especially done the right way! I spend only three to four minutes a day on my abdominals!

I start with Hit the Spot abs because your abdominals are the core—the center of your body. These muscles are responsible for maintaining good posture and protect most of your vital organs. Plus, more fat around your middle—closest to your heart—increases the chance of heart disease. The risk of colon cancer is twice as high in men who don't exercise; having a large waist (more than 43 inches) doubles the risk. Strong abdominals are a must! Don't be discouraged if you only can do a couple of reps the first few times you try these exercises. Most people find abdominal work very difficult for a couple of reasons. First, and most commonly, their abdominal and lower back regions are in terrible shape. Second, the only movement that remotely mimics the ab crunch is getting out of bed. Most of us only get out of bed once a day, so our muscles aren't trained to repeat that motion several times in a row.

AB TIPS

ABS Here are a few very important things that you should know about doing abdominal exercises to make them as safe and effective as possible:

1. **It is critical that you keep your lower back pressed firmly to the floor throughout the movement. Feel as though you are pressing your navel flat into your spine.**

2. **Never pull on your head during the movement. This can put unnecessary strain on your neck and upper back. Always *rest* your head in your hands and keep your chin up. I like to tell people to imagine an orange under their chins. If you look too far up it will fall out, look too far down and you'll squeeze the juice out of the orange.**

3. **I can't tell you how many times over the years people have confessed to me that they do tons of crunches but they still have tummies that stick out. Here's a little secret to guarantee that you get the greatest flattening effect from your crunches. When you are in the crunching phase of the exercise, it is *imperative* that you exhale! If you do your ab work with a diaphragm full of air, you'll build a hard tummy that actually sticks out. No kidding. Just making sure that you exhale as you come up with each rep**

means the difference between a hard, round tummy or a flat, sexy tummy.

Practice right now proper breathing during a crunch:

- **Lie on your back, bend your knees and place your hands on your tummy.**

- **Inhale and slowly fill your diaphragm with air—your hands should be lifting as if your tummy is inflating a balloon.**

- **Now, slowly raise up your head and shoulders (crunching) and exhale all the air, deflating, flattening your tummy, letting all the air out of that balloon, navel to spine hollow. That's how you breathe during each sit-up (crunch).**

- **Slower is better when doing sit-ups—use the muscle, not momentum.**

- **Only come halfway up. There's no sense in coming all the way up, since once you go past a 45-degree angle you are no longer using your abs, but may be straining your back.**

Do you have a bulging belly? Then it's crunch time. No more beer bellies. Trouble is, too many pounds at the waist can wreak havoc with the back.

Poor posture and weak abdominals also can make the belly bulge. Get a firm, flat, sexy stomach. In 21 days you can sculpt your stomach muscles and learn everything you need to know to get the flattest, firmest stomach.

YOU CAN DO THESE AB EXERCISES WHILE USING YOUR ABCOACH (AB-ROLLING PRODUCT). IT'S A GREAT COMPLEMENT TO YOUR WORKOUT.

I have been described on TV talk shows as having the hardest stomach in America. A rock-hard tummy has been my trademark for years. I have had more people than I can count feel my tummy—everyone from Bryant Gumbel to Jay Leno to Regis and Kathie Lee, Dustin Hoffman to Martina Navratilova to David Robinson to Colin Powell to CEOs all over the world, even the then-President of the United States, George Bush.

The following Hit the Spot ab exercises are the best ones for targeting all parts of the tummy region. We will be working the entire *rectus abdominus*—the muscle that runs vertically from the chest bone (*sternum*) going all the way down to the pelvic bone. We will also zero in on the internal and external oblique muscles—the sides and front of your waistline (no more middle-age spread and no more love handles).

And another important problem area for most of us is . . . below the belly button. The lower tummy is the hardest area to target. It is the least used of the three abdominal muscles in daily activity. If you've had a baby, abdominal surgery, or a C-section, it can be especially hard to re-educate those muscles. Having had two babies myself, I know it can be difficult, but I recovered the rock-hard stomach I'm famous for. I went from a 44-inch waistline (9 months pregnant) to a 24-inch waist in three months. I will teach you the key exercises I did to target the lower tummy.

Now you can choose to do all of these for a great variety or just do one or two. I always do one for the entire front (crunches), one for the obliques (oblique curls) and one for the lower tummy (reverse sit-up). It only takes me a few minutes a day to maintain my rock-hard tummy.

HOW MANY: With each ab exercise begin with one set of 8–12 reps and gradually progress to two sets of 8–12 reps. The most important part of doing your ab exercises is proper form. Don't cheat!

WHEN YOU'LL SEE RESULTS: Do three of these ab exercises at least four days a week and you will see a noticeable improvement in three weeks. Remember it's a three-prong attack: aerobic/cardio workouts, eating right, and ab work.

MY AB SECRETS:

- **It is extremely important to be aware of good posture all day long—having good posture helps retrain those muscles in the stomach that can sag and bulge if we forget about them.**

- **Remember, focus on the quality of each crunch, not the quantity!**

- **Another key technique is visualization—pull in your tummy throughout the day. Make believe that someone is going to punch you in the stomach. Contract your abdominal mus-**

cles and hold them for ten seconds: That is equal to one sit-up! You can be sitting at your desk, or in your car or watching TV, while you are toning and tightening your abs without ever getting down on the floor.

- Don't forget to isolate those muscles properly, using extreme precision. Slower is always better in ab work!

CRUNCHES

ABS This is one of the key exercises for working on the entire front of your tummy (rectus abdominus). If you're only going to do one abdominal exercise, do this one. It can be done by everyone regardless of their beginning level of fitness. The movement is easy to do and puts absolutely no strain on your lower back. Remember, when doing these as well as the other abdominal exercises, your form is very important, so read the instructions carefully.

- **Lie on your back with your knees bent and your feet on the floor (as shown).**

- **Press your lower back firmly into the floor. There should be no arch in your back at all.**

- **Rest your head in your hands but keep your neck and shoulders relaxed.**

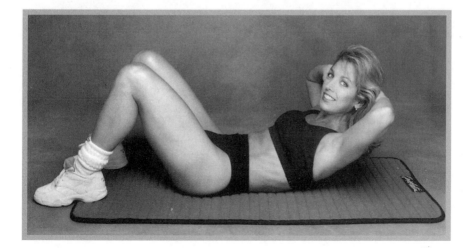

- **Tighten and contract your abdominal and slowly lift your shoulders off the floor.**

- **EXHALE AS YOU CRUNCH!**

- **Slowly lower your shoulders to the floor and repeat.**

- **Watch your form.**

- **Make sure your abs stay tight throughout the exercise.**

- **Don't do these quickly; keep slow and focused.**

It's your choice . . . Once you've conquered the basic crunch, try my variations. Challenge yourself!

VARIATIONS

Level 2 Crunch— *Intermediate*

Same as the basic crunch, but hands are crossed in front.

- **Use your abs to roll yourself up.**

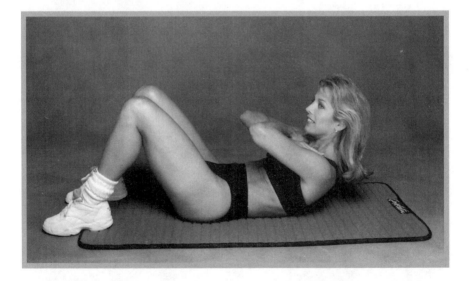

- **Pause at the top of movement, then lower yourself back to the starting position.**

Level 3 Crunch—*Advanced*

Same as the crunch, but arms are extended parallel to your body.

- **Use your abs to reach your hands to your knees.**

- **Pulse up.**

- **Lower your shoulders, allowing your blades to lightly touch the floor.**

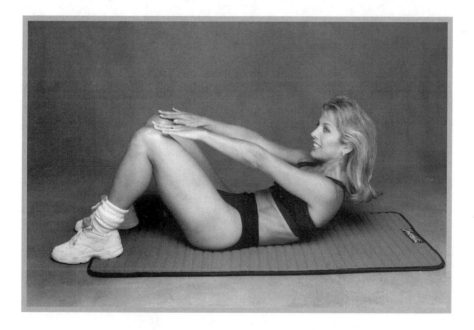

MID-SECTION MIRACLES
AB MUSCLES ARE LIKE A GIRDLE —
THEY'LL KEEP YOUR STOMACH IN . . . FLAT.

Level 4 Crunch—*Advanced*

Same as crunch, but arms are extended in an inverted "V" overhead.

- **Allow head to rest on upper arms.**

- **Use abs to raise torso toward knees.**

- **In a controlled motion, lower torso to starting position.**

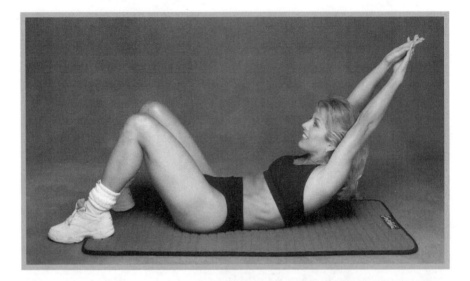

The Rope Climb Crunch—*Challenge*

Same as the crunch, but legs are extended straight up (knees unlocked).

- **Arms extended up.**

- **Use abs to lift torso.**

- **Next, use abs to further elevate torso as hands mimic a rope-climbing motion.**

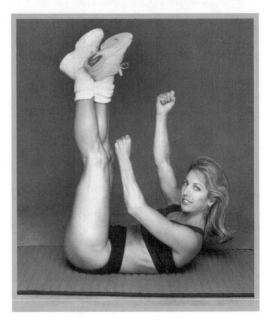

The Comfort Crunch (with chair)

Lie flat on your back, thighs perpendicular to your body, knees together and legs extended, resting on a chair.

- **Use abs to slowly lift forehead toward your knees.**

- **Keep constant tension on the abs throughout the entire range of motion.**

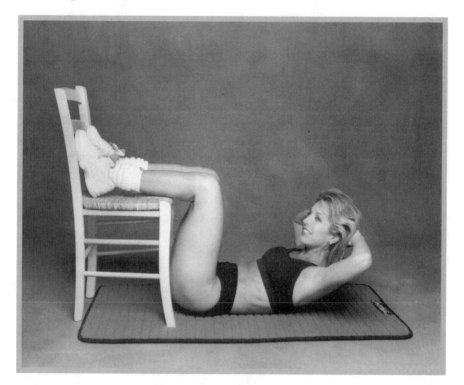

LAUGH, LAUGH HARD—
YOU'RE TONING YOUR TUMMY!

LOWER-TUMMY TIGHTENERS

This is by far the most effective exercise for your lower abdominal region. Although it works the entire ab region, it really isolates the lower abs. Of course, the lower abdominals are not a separate muscle, but the *rectus abdominus* is a very long muscle, and when the pelvis is moved upward during the exercise, the lower portion does the work. This is the perfect solution for any woman who has had a baby, particularly via a c-section.

- **Lie on the floor, and place your hands palms down just beneath your buttocks. This allows you to keep your lower back flat on the floor during the exercise.**

- **Lift your legs off the floor, bend them slightly and cross your ankles.**

- **Exhale as you lift your bent knees toward your chest. Your knees should stay bent at the same angle throughout the exercise.**

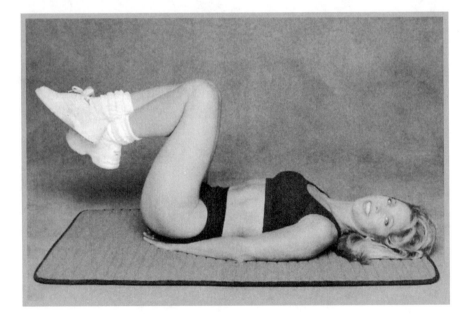

- Lower your legs slightly back down and repeat.

- Initiate this movement by first contracting the lower abs.

- This is a very short range of movement: your tailbone should lift off the floor only three to five inches.

- Do not swing your legs!

- Watch your form!

VARIATIONS

Lower Tummy Controller—*Beginner*

- Place a towel between your knees.

- Lift your hips up so pelvis is tilted and buttocks are off the floor a few inches.

- Relax, then repeat 8–12 reps.

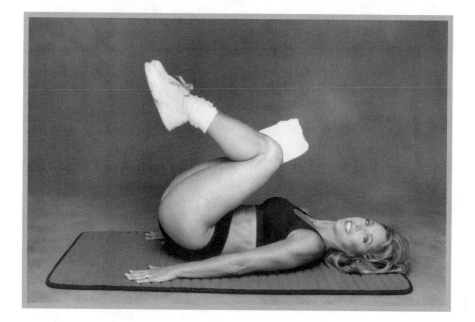

Lower Tummy Flattener—*Intermediate*

- Place a towel between your knees and feel more lower abs and inner thighs working. . . . It helps to "zero in" on the muscles closest to the pelvic bone. Challenge yourself by keeping your legs straight.

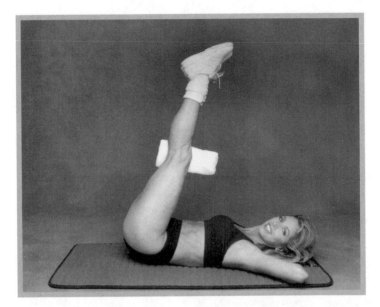

Lower Tummy Firmer—*Advanced*

- Straight legs, feet flexed and turned out, lift feet up as though you are placing footprints on the ceiling.

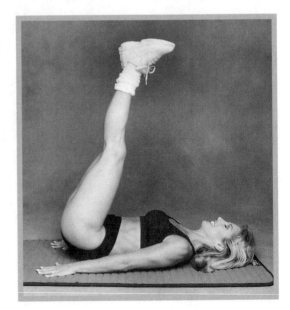

OBLIQUE CURLS

This exercise is almost identical to our first tummy-tightening crunch exercise. The only difference is that we are only going to raise one shoulder blade off the floor at a time. By doing so, you are able to focus on the internal and external obliques on the side of your tummy that support you laterally. As with all of our ab exercises, be sure that you try to contract your muscles with every rep. These are great waistline whittlers that will help get rid of those love handles we all hate.

- **Lie on the floor and cross your left foot over your right knee.**

- **Press your back firmly into the floor. There should be no arch in your back at all.**

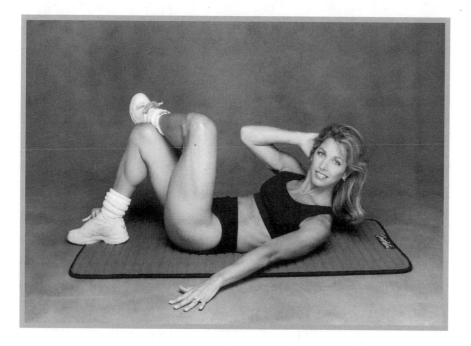

- **Place your left hand out to your side and your right hand behind your head.**

- **Exhale as you lift your left shoulder blade off the floor. You're not going to actually touch your elbow to your opposite knee, just move in that direction.**

- As soon as you have finished the reps on this side, repeat the same movement for the other side by switching the positions of your hands and your feet.

VARIATIONS

Waistline Trimmer

- Place towel between knees, squeezing together and slightly tilting legs to the side. Do 8–12 crunches, then repeat crunches on the other side of the waist by simply shifting your knees to the other side.

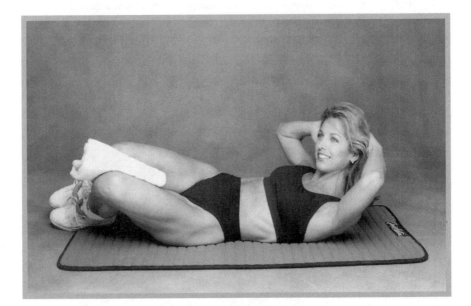

GET A TRIM, SLIM WAISTLINE
WE'LL SHRINK MIDDLE-AGE SPREAD

Waistline Slimmer

- Begin as shown in photo with left leg extended and right elbow bent. Bend and pull knee toward elbow and feel the "crunch." Switch sides.

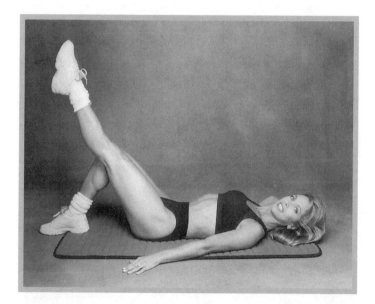

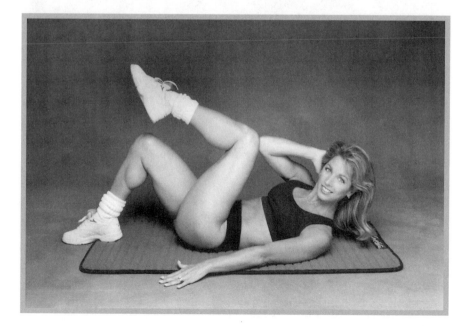

BICYCLES

This exercise is a little more difficult to do because it involves most of the abdominal region. By moving both the arms and the legs at the same time, you involve the upper and lower regions of your tummy. It's pretty easy to lose control of the form on this one, so really concentrate! Think belly button in, lower back pressed into floor, flat hollow stomach.

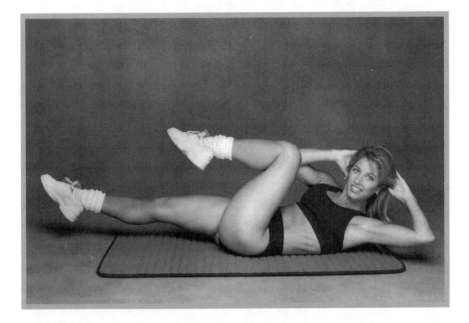

- **Lie on the floor with your right leg straight and your left knee bent.**

- **Press your back firmly into the floor—there should be no arch in it at all.**

- **Rest your head in your hands, but keep your neck and shoulders relaxed.**

- **Exhale as you pull your right knee in toward your chest. At the same time, raise your left shoulder to meet your right knee.**

- **Straighten out the right leg. As you do, draw the left leg to your chest, meeting it with your elbow.**

- **Continue to alternate side to side, simulating riding a bicycle.**

- **Watch your form.**

- **Keep the movement smooth and flowing, and try to keep your feet and shoulders from touching the floor.**

MODIFICATIONS: If you find that the bicycles are too difficult, try these three easier ones. Just be sure to keep the lower back pressed into the floor and pull your abdomen in toward your spine.

VARIATIONS

Total Ab Sculptor— *Beginner*

- **Bend knees, alternating "toe taps" to floor.**

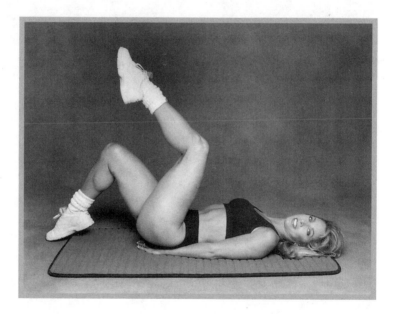

Total Ab Trimmer—*Intermediate*

- **Hands under hips and head and shoulders up.**

- **Alternate legs repeatedly.**

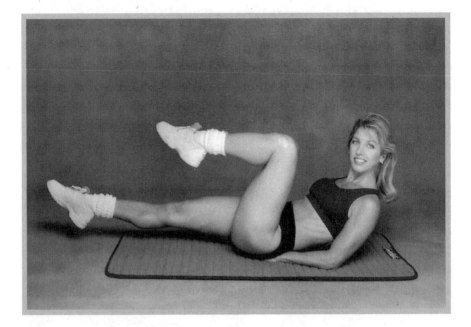

Total Ab Slimmer—*Advanced*

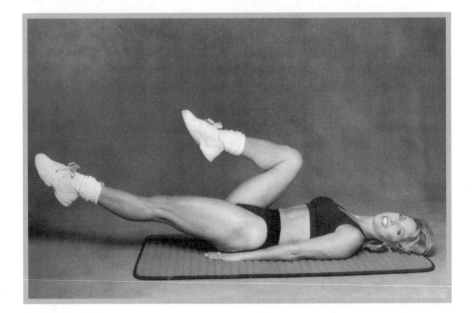

- **Relax your upper body and place hands under hips.**

- **Very important that you press lower back into floor.**

- **Alternate legs repeatedly.**

ROCK-HARD ABS

This is an extremely challenging exercise—very advanced—from my gymnastics days. It is essential that your abs and back are strong to support the movement. I like to do this one to intensify and maximize my ab workout, and get those washboard abs! But I do only one set of 8–12 reps.

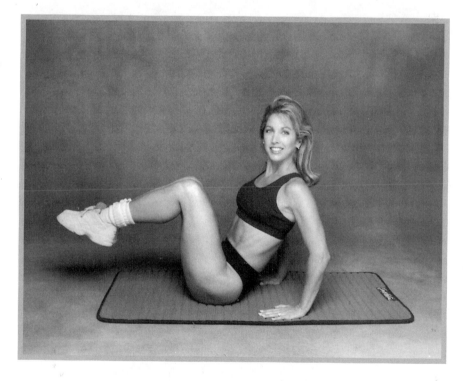

- **Sit on the floor, placing your hands on the floor next to you. For support, lean back slightly, bending your elbows.**

- **Bend your knees and bring them in toward your chest, raising your feet off the floor.**

- Extend your legs straight out in front of you, using your abs to keep them off the floor and to control the movement. It's important to keep your abs tight throughout the entire movement.

- Pull your legs back into your chest, then extend them again.

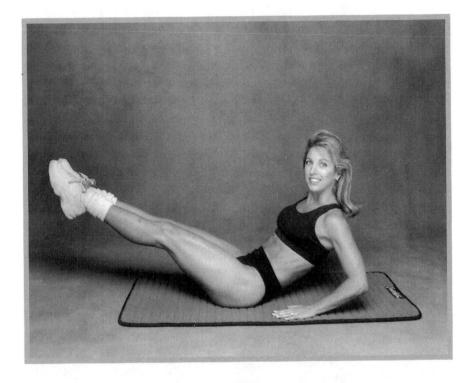

TO PREVENT BELLY BLOATEDNESS:
- DON'T CHEW GUM
- DON'T SIP FROM A STRAW
- DON'T DRINK TOO MANY CARBONATED BEVERAGES
- EAT SLOWLY

Ab Definer

- **For obliques, and to really see great definition and a smaller waistline, slant your body to the side and tuck in and out slowly.**

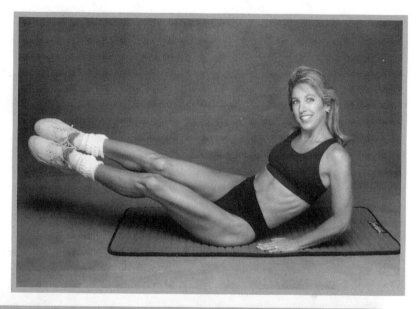

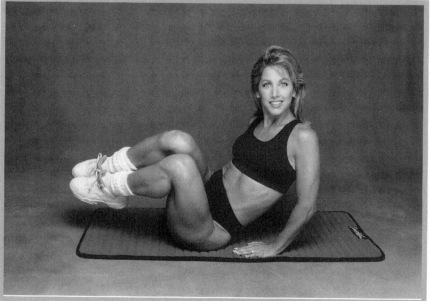

- **Hold stretches 15–30 seconds.**

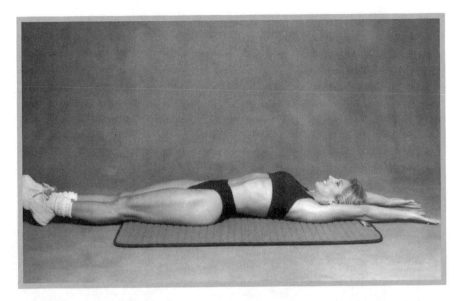

- **Abdominal cool down.**

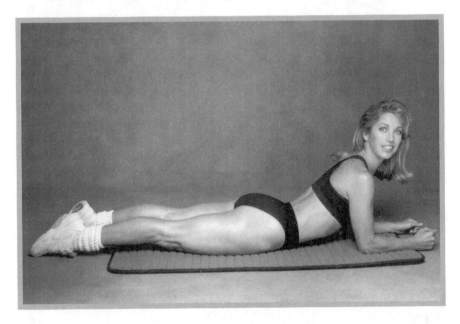

- **Full-body stretch.**

HIPS AND THIGHS

DEAR DENISE,

*Thanks to your Hit the Spot exercises I have lost 30 pounds!
I have gone from a size 24 to an 18, lost inches around my hips . . .
and plan to lose more!*

TONYA—NEW MEXICO

DEAR DENISE,

*I am 37 and had four children in the span of six years. I also have a
very sedentary job (I am a piano teacher), so I didn't get much
exercise. Needless to say, this took a toll on my body. Last summer,
however, I started working out and following your advice for eating
a low-fat diet and not eating late at night. I lost 41 pounds, going
from a size 14 to a size 8! Your tapes and books are wonderful for
those of us that are not particularly athletic. I never felt that your
exercises were too difficult to manage. Whenever anyone asks how I
did it, I always reply: my personal trainer—Denise Austin!*

LORI—BETHESDA, MARYLAND

DEAR DENISE,

*Thanks to your Hit the Spot thigh exercises I lost one inch in each
thigh in just one month! I am 45 years old and for the first time I
share clothes with my teenage daughter!*

LISA—TAMPA, FLORIDA

The biggest problem areas for most women are their hips and thighs. This is rooted in biology: Women of childbearing years store most of their body fat in these areas. But don't despair, the good news is that fat deposits on the hips and thighs are easily burned. Why? Because the large muscle groups of the body burn calories more efficiently.

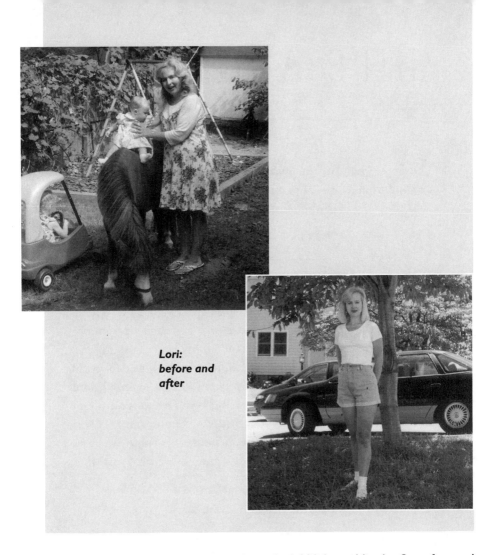

Lori:
before and
after

If this is your problem spot, you're in luck. With my Hit the Spot focused exercise plan, we can resize your thighs and change the shape and contour of your lower body.

Cellulite—that dreaded cottage-cheese look—is the upper layer of fat that lies between connective-tissue fibers that attach muscle to skin. Cellulite is just fat on top of fat. Excess fat pushing through the weakened skin fibers forms a web around the fat, causing cellulite, just like your mattress bulges between the stitching. This is why the skin gets lumpy and dimpled. Cellulite is mainly caused by lack of muscle tone.

All these exercises will zero in and redefine your hips and thighs. I don't know anybody who doesn't want shapely thighs, free of cellulite! We'll concentrate on your inner thighs (no more jigglies), your outer thighs (no more saddlebags), the back of your thighs (for a great rear view) and we'll also slim

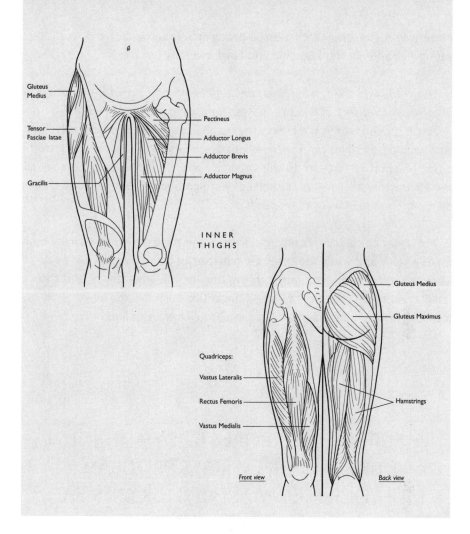

Gluteus Medius

Tensor Fasciae latae

Gracilis

Pectineus

Adductor Longus

Adductor Brevis

Adductor Magnus

INNER THIGHS

Gluteus Medius

Gluteus Maximus

Quadriceps:

Vastus Lateralis

Rectus Femoris

Vastus Medialis

Hamstrings

Front view   *Back view*

those hips. Give me your lower half for just minutes a day and we will make it your better half—instantly!

A word here about thigh creams. Creams can improve the appearance of your skin, but they do not change muscles or the shape of your body. A cellulite cream used in conjunction with exercise can make a small difference, but don't rely on the cream alone.

Many women have resorted to liposuction and achieved positive results. However, I am not in favor of such extreme measures. With the right eating habits and toning exercises, you can see dramatic results in a short time! We'll spot train your thighs and slenderize your hips to a sexy, lean size. You will lose inches from your hips and thighs, and get the shape you want.

WHEN YOU'LL SEE RESULTS: You'll see an improvement in as little as three weeks. Remember, it's a three-prong attack: aerobic/cardio workouts, eating well and Hit the Spot Hip and Thigh exercises.

HOW MANY: With each exercise, begin with one set of 8–12 reps and progress to two sets of 8–12 reps. Rest for 15 seconds between sets.

I recommend that you increase the number of repetitions gradually. Your goal should be to aim for 16–24 repetitions every time you do these exercises. As soon as you can do this relatively easily, add the second set of all the exercises with weights (either holding dumbbells, a bar on your shoulders or using ankle weights or bands).

HOW OFTEN: Try to complete four of the thigh exercises at least four times a week and you'll see results in a matter of three weeks. I like to do at least one exercise for the outer thighs, one for the inner thighs and then a couple that really target the hips and the entire thigh, like the lunge or squat. It only takes a few minutes. . . . Go for it! You'll have lean legs.

BE SURE TO USE PROPER BODY ALIGNMENT
DURING YOUR EXERCISE PROGRAM.
KEEP YOUR ELBOW AND KNEE JOINTS SAFE
BY NOT LOCKING THEM.

LUNGES

If the only exercises you did for your legs were lunges, your legs would look terrific! This is one of the most effective exercises you can do to work the *entire* leg. Lunges can be done with no weights at all, while holding dumbbells or with a bar on your shoulders. It is a difficult exercise, so start without any weight. After you do add weights, increase their size gradually.

- **Start with one foot in front of the other as though you are taking a giant step (chair optional for balance).**

- **Lower yourself, bending both knees, but make sure your knee stays in line with your ankle. Try not to bang your back knee on the floor.**

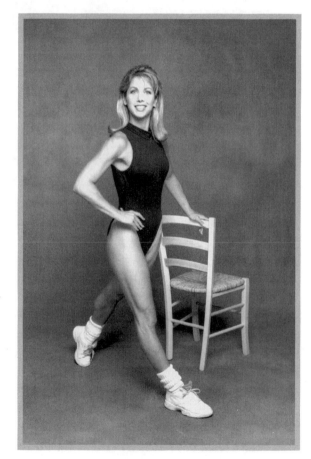

- **Your weight should be on your back toes and on your front heel.**

- **Straighten legs until you are standing, and lower yourself again. Do 16–24 reps.**

- **Repeat with opposite leg.**

- **Watch your form.**

- **Keep your back straight.**

- **Don't let your front knee extend over the front of your toes.**

- **If you have bad knees, modify this lunge and only bend your knees slightly—you're still firming those thighs!**

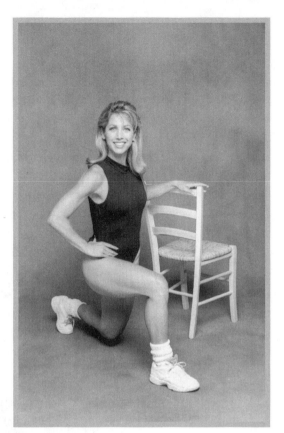

SQUATS

Thighs This is another great leg exercise for the legs and is one of my favorites. It works *three* different muscle groups: the *quadriceps* (front of the leg), the *hamstrings* (back of the leg) and the *gluteals* (the muscles in your buttocks). It is helpful to elevate your heels a bit (place a book under your heels) to help you with your balance. You can use dumbbells once you get the hang of it.

- **Stand with your feet a little wider than your hips. Standing in front of a chair will guide you into the right position.**

- **Your back should be straight and your abs tight.**

- **Place your hands on your hips. If you're using weights, hands are at your shoulders.**

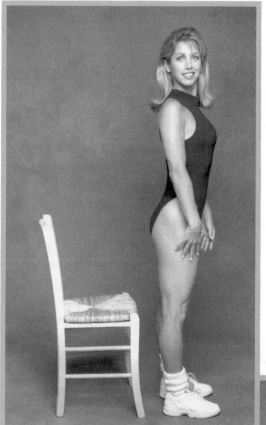

- Bend your knees and begin to squat. As you start your movement, raise your hands in front of you as shown in the picture. This will help your balance. Go as low as you comfortably can (never past a 90-degree angle), then stand back up.

- Feel as though you are sitting back, with your body's weight in your heels.

- Do this one in front of a mirror, using the chair, until you get the hang of it.

- Watch your form.

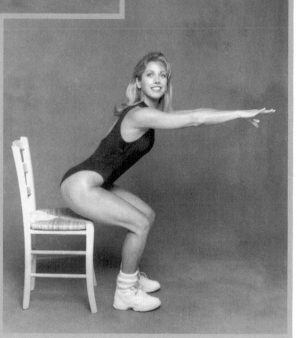

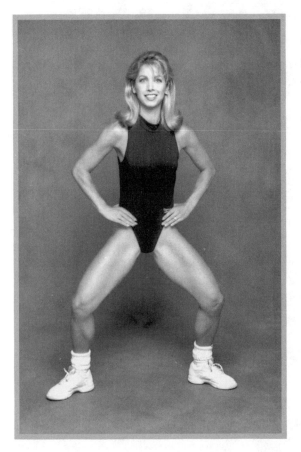

The Wide-Stance Squat
—*Intermediate*

• Same as the squat but with a wide stance. Your feet are slightly turned out, like second position in ballet, to put extra emphasis on the inner thighs and buttocks.

THE GREAT FEELING OF SUCCESS RESULTS FROM DOING IT YOURSELF. I BELIEVE MOTIVATION FOLLOWS AFTER YOU BECOME A BIT SUCCESSFUL. YOU REALIZE THAT FROM YOUR OWN EFFORTS YOU HAVE MADE A DIFFERENCE . . . YOU FEEL GOOD ABOUT YOURSELF!

OUTER-THIGH TRIMMER

No more saddlebags! This is a terrific exercise for your outer thighs. You can do this one anytime, anywhere, standing up or lying down. You'll want to start this exercise using no weights. Gradually add more resistance by strapping on ankle weights or by using a resistance-type elastic band. As you do this exercise, be sure that you don't swing your leg—move deliberately and really concentrate on the outer part of your thigh.

- **Lie on the floor with your left side down. Your head, shoulders, and hips should all be aligned.**

- **Bend your left leg behind you and put your right hand down in front of you for balance.**

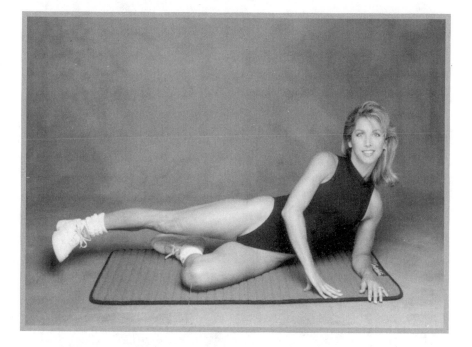

- **Keeping your right leg straight and your foot relaxed, slowly raise your leg. Lower it back to the floor, then repeat. You can use ankle weights to challenge yourself.**

- This is a very short movement, so be careful not to raise your leg too high. You should be focusing on the outer thigh of the top leg.

- After you have completed 16–24 reps, turn over and repeat the exercise on the other leg.

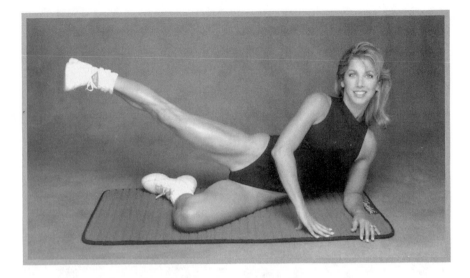

VARIATIONS

The Comfort Thigh Raise—*Beginner*

- Same as outer-thigh raise, but rest your head on a pillow for perfect alignment.

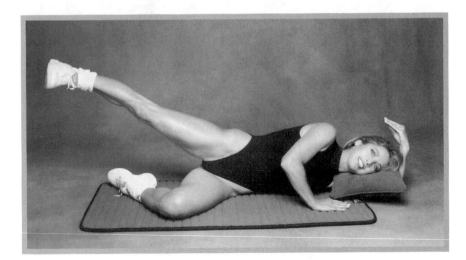

The Outer-Thigh Shaper

- **Same motion as outer-thigh raise, but try standing up (chair optional).**

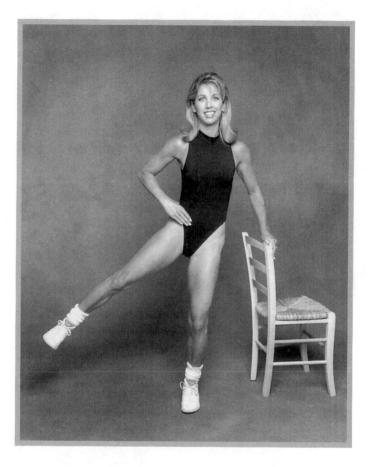

IF YOU REST..YOU'LL RUST!

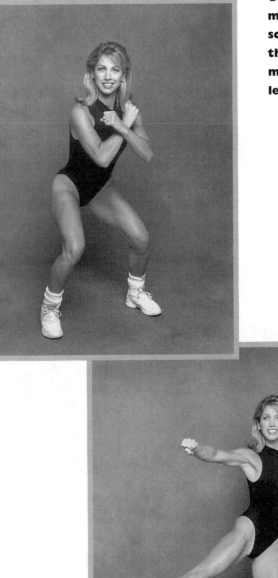

- **Combines the motions of a squat and outer-thigh raise—you may alternate legs.**

INNER-THIGH FIRMER

The inner thighs are one of the most underused muscles of the body. Even when you walk or run, you're still not targeting them. That's why you must position your body to zero in on those inner thighs and flabby knees. These are the best exercises to firm, tone and tighten those rubbing thighs. No more jigglies!

- **Lie on the floor with your left side down. Your head, shoulders and hips should all be aligned. Resting your head on a pillow is the best way to achieve proper form.**

- **Bend your right leg and place it on the floor in front of you for balance.**

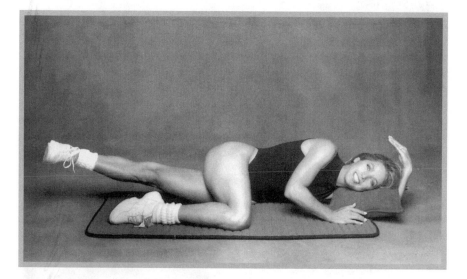

- **Keeping your left leg straight and your foot flexed, slowly raise your leg. Lower it back to the floor, then repeat.**

- **This is a very short movement, so be careful not to raise your leg too high. You should be focusing on the outer thigh of your top leg.**

- **Your left foot should remain flexed and parallel to the floor throughout the movement.**

- **After you have completed your two sets (16–24 reps), turn over and repeat the exercise on the opposite leg.**

The Inner-Thigh Tightener—*Advanced*

- **Frog position. Lie on your back and place towel under buttocks. To keep back in alignment, slowly lower legs, pressing soles of your feet together. Continue small presses up and down.**

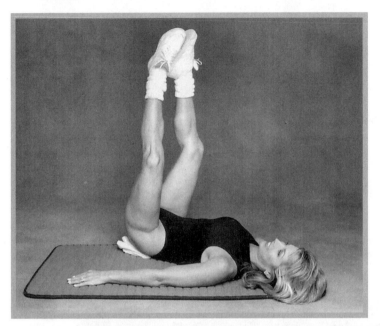

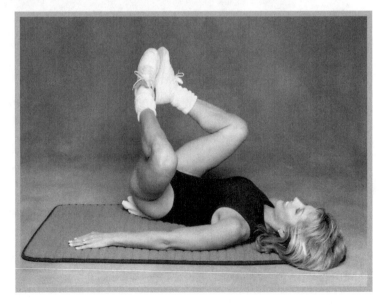

The Inner-Thigh Toner

- **Standing (chair optional) inner-thigh sweep over standing leg.**

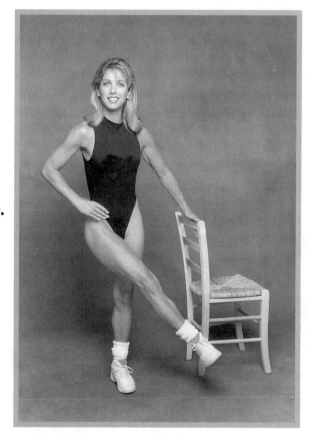

BEST KEPT THIGH SECRET:
WHENEVER YOU'RE GOING UP STAIRS,
SKIP A STEP—"DOUBLE-UP." YOU'LL
GET FIRM, DEFINED THIGHS FAST!

BACK-OF-THIGH FIRMER

Thighs

Inactivity causes muscles to lose their tone. Since most of us sit for at least seven and one-half hours a day, we begin to get what I call *seatitis*. . . . and can just feel our hips and thighs spreading. Here are some great ways to firm, shape and trim the backs of your thighs.

- **Kneel on the floor with your elbows and hands on the floor.**

- **Be sure to keep your back flat, abs tight and your hips square to the floor.**

- **Raise one leg off the floor, keeping it straight.**

- **Slowly raise your leg up and down, squeezing your buttocks (16–24 reps).**

- **Switch legs and repeat.**

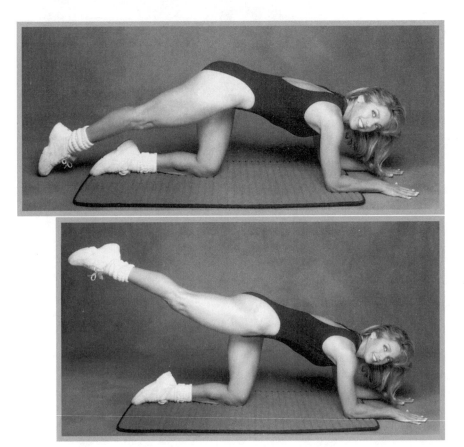

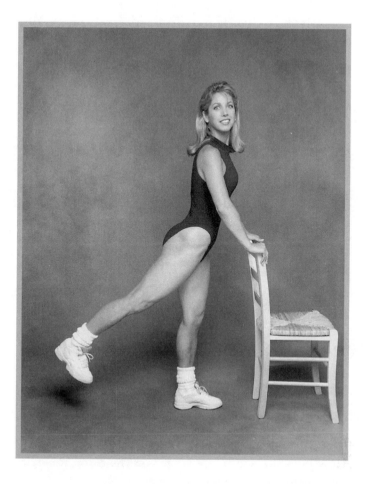

Thigh Sculptor, Standing

- **Stand and lift leg to back. Squeeze your buttocks and concentrate on keeping abs tight. Don't arch the lower back! (Use a chair for balance.)**

HAMSTRING CURLS

Thighs

Do you want shapely thighs without the flab? Do you want to walk around the pool without a towel wrapped around your waist? These exercises truly zero in on the backs of your thighs, firming and sculpting them. No more cellulite!

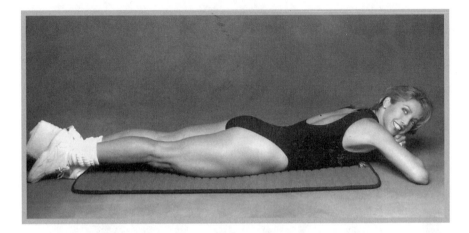

- **Lie on your stomach.**

- **Place a folded towel between your feet, keeping your legs straight.**

- **Keeping your pelvis and thighs on the floor, slowly curl your heels toward your buttocks.**

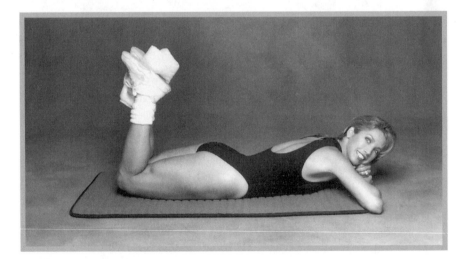

- Be sure to really squeeze your buttocks together throughout the entire movement.

- Lower your legs to the starting position and repeat the
  exercise. You should feel this in the back of your thighs.

VARIATIONS

The Hamstring Sculptor—*Intermediate*

- In a kneeling position, with one thigh parallel to the floor,
  slowly bend your knee, then straighten. Keep abs strong.
  Don't arch your back.

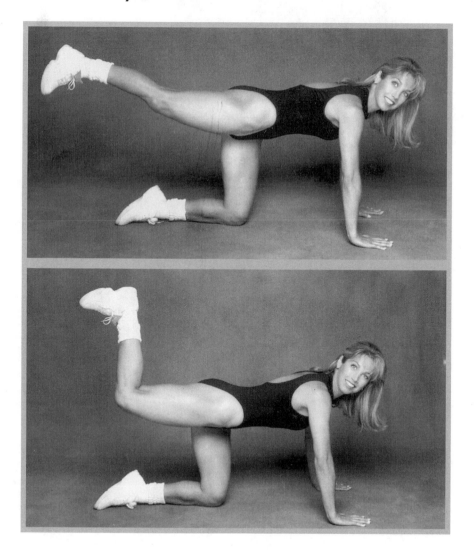

The Rear-View Lifter—*Standing position hamstring curl*

- **Heel toward buttocks, back straight and abs tight.**

- **You can add ankle weights if you like.**

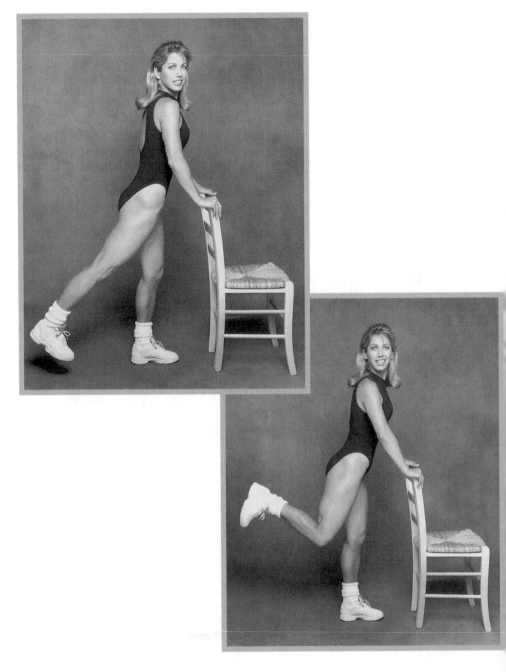

QUAD TONER

Thighs These exercises are designed to firm, tone and tighten the front of your thighs. These leg extensions will give you the most definition in your thighs. You'll look great in your shorts . . . and short skirts! These are also the perfect exercises to strengthen all the muscles surrounding your knee to help prevent knee injuries. Great to get you ready for skiing. Add 1–2 pound ankle weights for quicker results.
No more saggy or flabby knees.

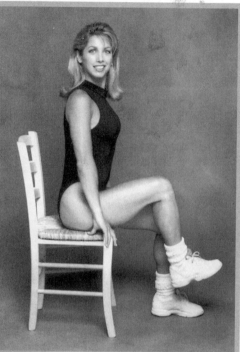

- Sit on chair with your back up straight and your abs tight.

- Raise your right foot off the floor, keeping your knee bent.

- Keeping your right foot flexed, slowly straighten your leg while tightening the top of your thigh.

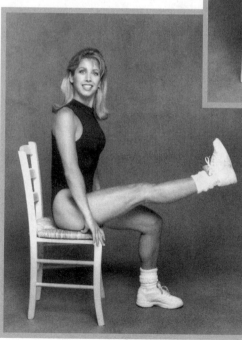

- Bend knee and repeat the movement.

- After you have completed one set of 8–12 reps, repeat the exercise with the alternate leg.

The Quad Shaper—*Beginner*

- Sit on floor. To make it easier, place your hands behind you. The farther forward you are, the harder it will be.

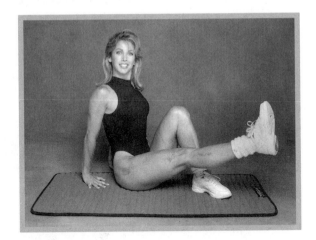

The Quad Sculptor—*Advanced*

- Standing leg extension.

- Bend and extend your leg. Use chair for support and balance.

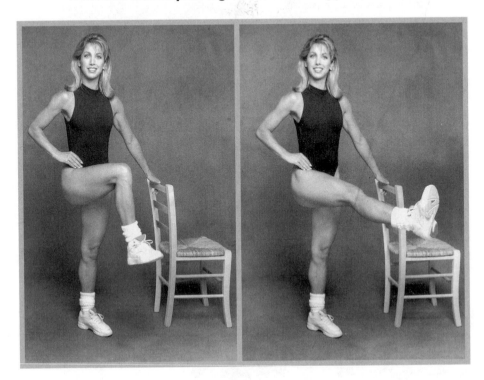

CALF SHAPER

Thighs

Do you want to give your hips and thighs a slimmer look? Then do my calf shaper. If you have some muscle, shape and form to the lower part of your leg, it will give more balance to your whole leg. Let's take, for instance, the bird-leg look. A skinny, bony lower leg can make the upper thigh look bigger and thicker. However, if you shape up and get some muscle definition in the lower leg, your upper thighs will appear smaller and better proportioned!

- **Place your hands on the back of a chair for balance.**

- **Lift your heels up and down slowly.**

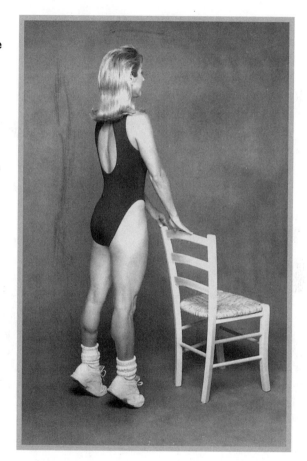

HIP
SLIMMER

Thighs

Hips are at the top of every woman's toughest-to-tackle list. They come in all shapes and sizes, but no matter what kind of hips you have, these hip shapers will get them slim, slim, slim. All these exercises will give you that sexy indentation on the side of your hip! You'll be eager to race to the pool to show it off!

- **Lie on your right side on a carpet or mat.**

- **Raise your torso and support yourself on your right forearm.**

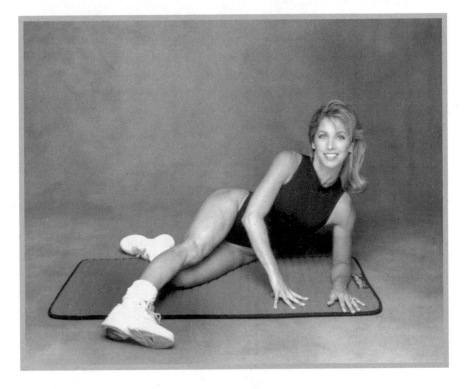

- **Bend your right leg back along the floor.**

- **Extend your left leg straight out to the front and flex the foot.**

- Raise your left foot 6 inches off the floor and slowly bring it down.

- Do 16-24 reps with left leg, then switch sides and repeat with right leg.

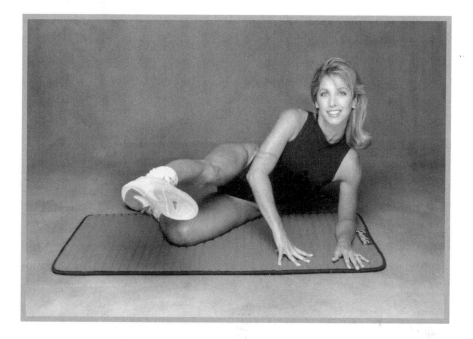

FOR GREAT LEGS: FORM A HABIT OF WALK-
ING EVERYWHERE YOU GO, IF POSSIBLE . . .
TO AND FROM WORK, AROUND THE BLOCK
INSTEAD OF A COFFEE BREAK.
YOU'LL GET MORE ENERGY.

The Outer-Hip Shaper—*Intermediate*

- Straighten both legs with one over the other.

- Do heel-toe with top leg. Touch your heel in front of your leg and then tap your toe behind your leg.

- Do 16-24 reps with this leg, then switch and repeat.

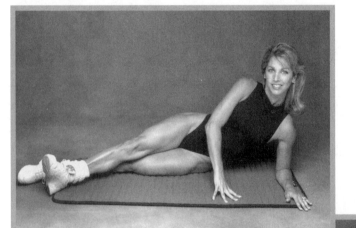

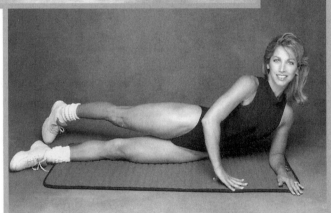

The Hip Toner—*Advanced*

- **Bent knee leg lift—hip over hip.**

- **Be sure to lift leg, ankle, knee and hip all together in one plane. Lift and lower top leg, 16-24 reps.**

- **Switch sides and repeat with other leg.**

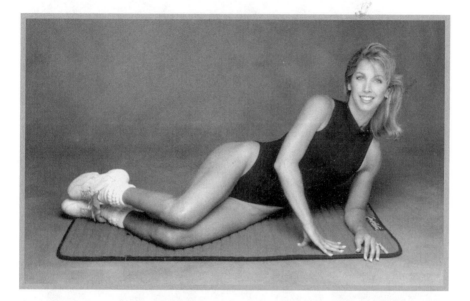

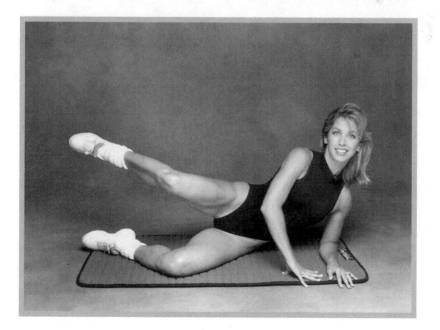

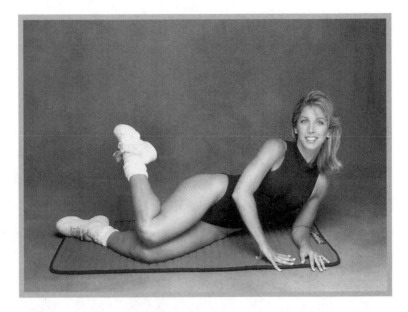

- **Knee touch, then leg extension. Be sure to keep abs tight and do not arch lower back!**

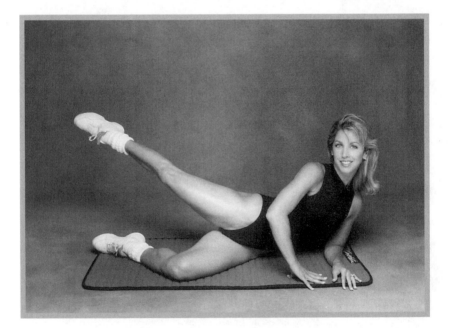

LOWER BODY
STRETCHES

- **Hold stretches for 15–30 seconds.**

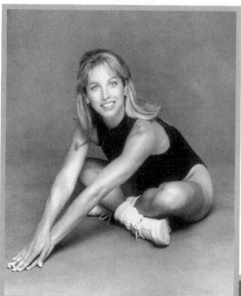

- **Hip-and-Thigh
  Stretch—
  Sit cross-legged and
  reach forward.**

- **Quad Stretch—
  Hold foot,
  gently pull
  heel toward
  buttocks and
  feel stretch in
  the front of
  your thighs.**

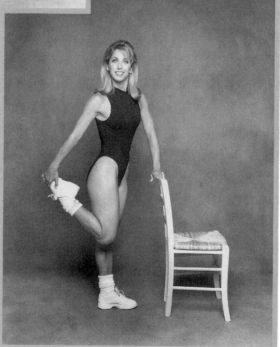

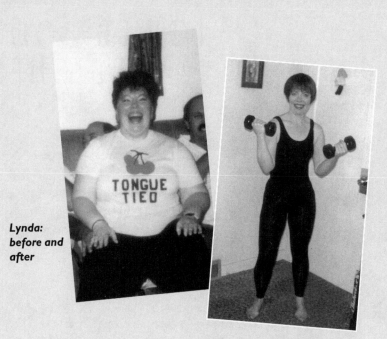

Lynda: before and after

Gluteus Minimus
(underneath Gluteus
Medius and Gluteus
Maximus)

Gluteus
Medius

Rotators

Gluteus
Maximus

BUNS

Squeeze your buttocks—anywhere, anytime—turn that idle time into toning time. When it comes to sculpting and tightening jiggly backsides my Hit the Spot Bun exercises are the best solution. To get results you need to focus on the quality, not the quantity, of the exercise! You can get a great rear view with any of these easy exercises that give your buttock muscles— your glutes—a lift! Do you want to look great from behind and feel sexy in jeans? Then try a few of these effective exercises for the best bun workout ever.

My Hit the Spot Buns routine has both standing and floor exercises. The standing ones target the *gluteus maximus* (the largest muscle located in the buns)! They help to tighten your derriere, lift your "cheeks" and work to create sexy hip indentations. My floor exercises zero in on the *gluteus medius* and *gluteus minimus* (two smaller muscles), and the *rotators* (six deep horizontal muscles). To make sure you use these muscles properly and get the maximum effect, work slowly and concentrate on each contraction!

HOW MANY: I recommend that you increase the number of repetitions gradually. Your goal is one set of 8–12 reps every time you do each bun exercise. As soon as you can do this with relative ease, add a second set (8–12 reps). Next, graduate to weights (3–5 pound hand weights or 1–2 pound ankle weights).

WHEN YOU'LL SEE RESULTS: Pick at least three of your favorite bun exercises, do them four days a week and you'll see a noticeable improvement in just three weeks. It will only take you a few minutes and you will have a fabulous derriere. A tighter tush.

Make the most of your bottom! Squeeze your buttock muscles as often as you can throughout the day—you can do this in line at the grocery store, in the car at a stoplight, even while watching TV!

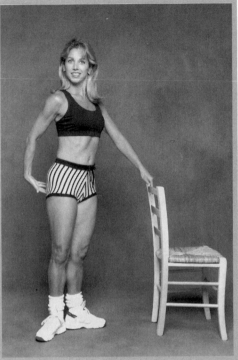

BOTTOMS UP

Buns

This is an easy exercise which will do wonders for the buns. . . . Just make sure you squeeze your buttocks. Feel as though you're squeezing that last drop of water out of a towel. A great bun burner!

- **Lie on your back, bend your knees and keep your feet flat on the floor.**

- **Extend your arms along your sides.**

- **Lift your buttocks off the floor (3–6 inches) by tilting your pelvis up, squeezing your buttocks and tightening your abdominals.**

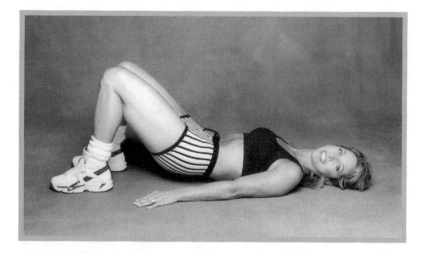

- **Hold for a few seconds and then lower your bottom down one vertebrae at a time. Repeat 8 times.**

VARIATIONS

The Glute Toner—*Advanced*

- **To add resistance, place right foot on left thigh. You will feel it more in the left cheek of the rear. Lift buns up and down 8-12 reps.**

- **Switch legs and repeat.**

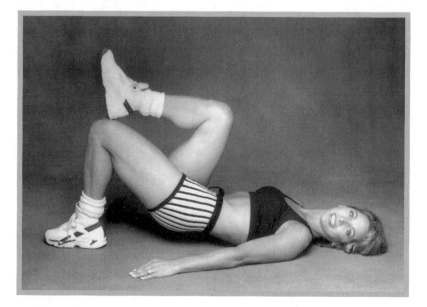

- **With legs straight out, press with arms to lift body off floor. Squeeze your buttock muscles for ten seconds. Relax and repeat twice.**

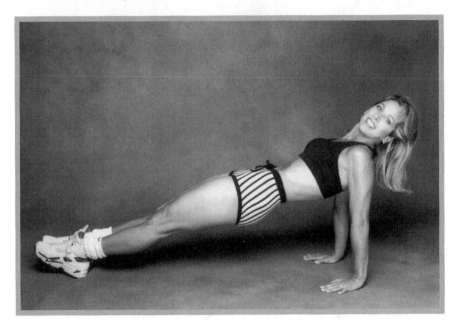

TUSH TIGHTENER

Buns This exercise will sculpt the buttocks. It actually will enhance your shape and appearance, giving you tight, rounded buns. Remember, when you leave a room, your backside is the last thing anyone sees!

- **Kneel on the floor with your elbows and hands on the floor.**

- **Be sure to keep your back flat, abs tight and your hips square to the floor.**

- **Raise your right leg off the floor, keeping it bent at a right angle. Thigh is parallel to the floor.**

- **Slowly raise your knee up and down, pressing your foot toward the ceiling, squeezing your buttocks.**

- **After you have completed the reps (16-24) with the right leg, repeat the exercise with the left leg.**

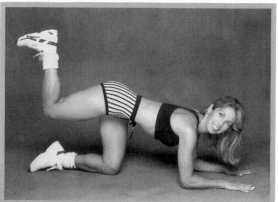

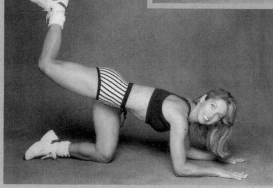

VARIATIONS

The Bun Burner—*Advanced*

- **On hands and knees and keeping hips square, cross bent knee over other leg.**

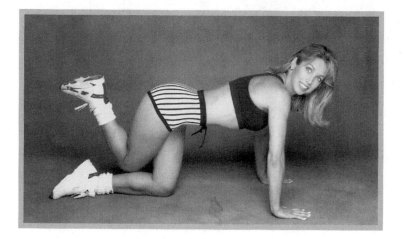

Bun Lifter—*Advanced*

- **On hands and knees, simultaneously extend right leg and left arm. Hold for 10 seconds, squeezing buns. Relax and repeat with the other leg.**

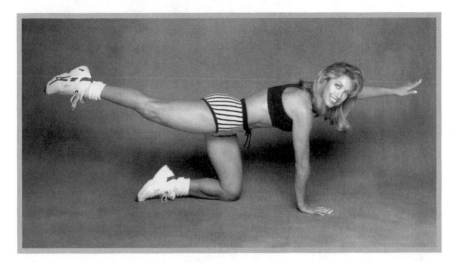

A Better Bottom

- **Stand up tall with your back straight and abs tight.**

- **Hold the chair for balance.**

- **Bend your right leg, keep foot flexed, and squeeze your buttocks. Heel toward rear end.**

- **Pulse the heel up 8-12 reps.**

- **Relax and switch legs.**

FANNY FIRMER

This exercise is great for the backs of your thighs and buttocks. Firm them up and look great in your jeans! Concentrate as you tighten and relax for maximum benefit.

- **Lie on your stomach with your arms folded under your chin and legs extended.**

- **Keep neck aligned. Lift right leg about 4–8 inches off the floor, anchoring your hips to the floor.**

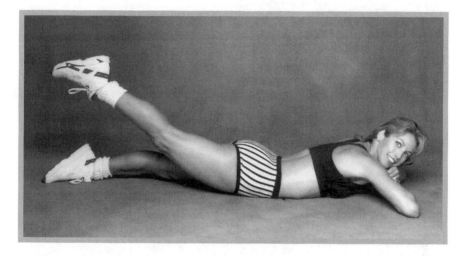

- **Squeeze your buttocks and concentrate on proper form; do not overarch your back.**

- **Hold for 10 seconds and relax.**

- **Repeat using opposite leg and hold for 10 seconds. Then repeat the whole sequence.**

THE ONLY WAY YOU WILL EVER CHANGE
YOUR SHAPE IS BY DEVELOPING MUSCLE.

BUTT TAPS

Buns

If I had to recommend just one lower body exercise, this would be it. Butt taps give the buttock muscles maximum-target tone action in a minimum amount of time. I love this one. I do it every day.

- **Stand with your feet a little wider than your hips. Your heels should be 3–6 inches from the seat of a chair.**

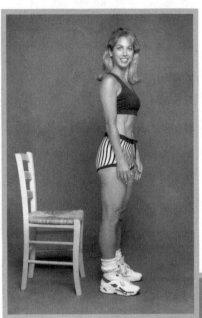

- **Your back is straight, abs are tight.**

- **Bend your knees and slowly lower yourself until your butt taps the chair. Be careful not to bounce!**

- **As soon as you tap the chair, straighten your legs and return to the starting position. Repeat the movement (8-12 reps).**

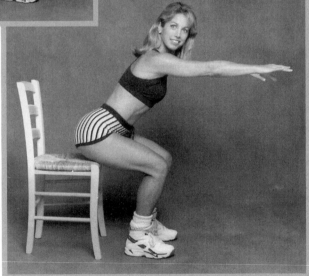

Wide-Leg Butt Taps
— Intermediate

- **Chair taps with wide stance and feet turned out.**

- **Great for thighs and buttocks.**

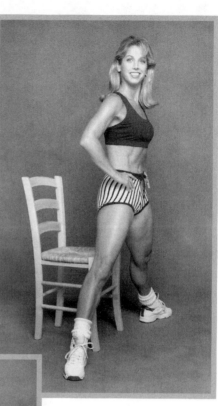

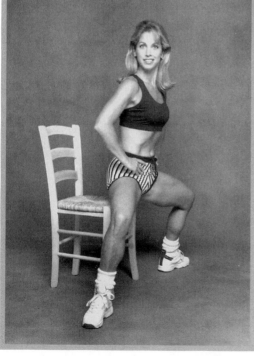

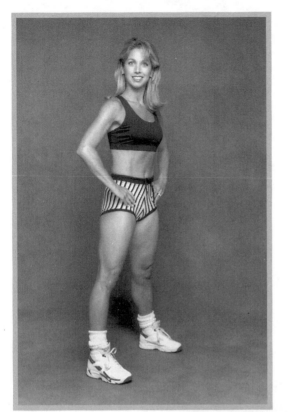

Basic Squat
- **Same as Butt Taps, without the chair. A little easier. I do this squat all the time, even while blow drying my hair.**

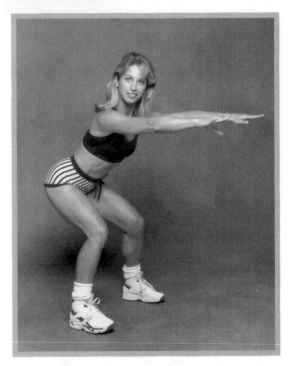

The Power Squats—*Advanced*

- **Squat with weights at hips.**

- **Squeeze the buttocks on the way up.**

- **Sit back with your body weight through your heels.**

- **If you have a history of knee problems, begin with a partial squat, one quarter of the way down.**

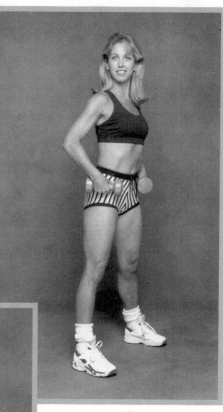

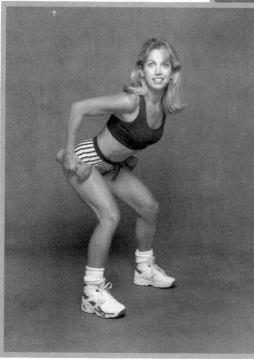

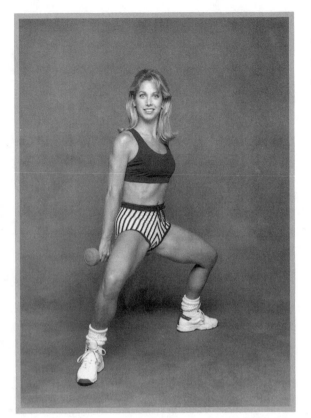

The Ultimate Squat
— Challenge

- **Wide stance with feet turned out and holding weights.**

- **Squeeze the buttocks on the way up.**

LUNGE DIPS

This move will trim the annoying bulges and flab you may find around your hips, thighs and buttocks. This one will definitely give your buttocks a lift, and help you look your best from behind.

- **Start with your feet about shoulder width apart. (You can use a chair back or counter for balance). Weights are optional.**

- **Place one foot forward.**

- **Bend your back knees and lower yourself toward the floor, so your tail bone moves straight down.**

- **Balancing your body weight over your front heel and your back toes, keep knees at 90 degree angles.**

- **Straighten your legs and raise yourself back up.**

- **Keeping your legs in the lunge position, repeat the dip's up and down movement, like an elevator. After you have completed one set (8–12 dips—down *and* up), alternate legs and repeat the exercise with the other leg.**

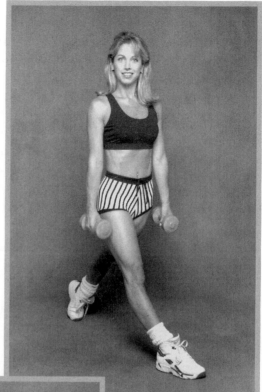

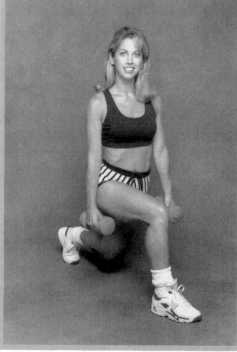

The Advanced Lunge

- **Using a step or bench, dip down and up in the lunge position. Make sure you push through the front heel. Weights are optional.**

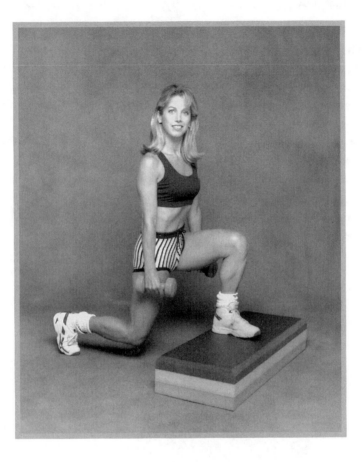

THINK ABOUT THE MUSCLE YOU ARE TONING AND IMAGINE IT GETTING FIRMER AND SLEEKER WITH EACH REP. . . .

BUTTOCKS STRETCHES

Buns

- **Hold** each stretch 15–30 seconds.

- **Best buns stretch—My favorite stretch for the buttocks and hamstrings.**

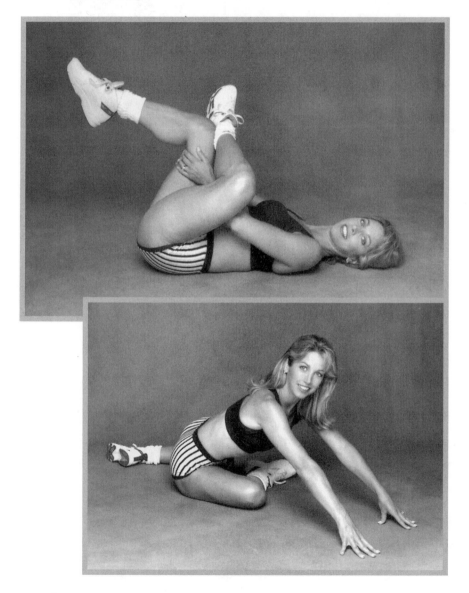

- **Cheek stretch—Lengthens the "cheek" of the front leg. Switch legs.**

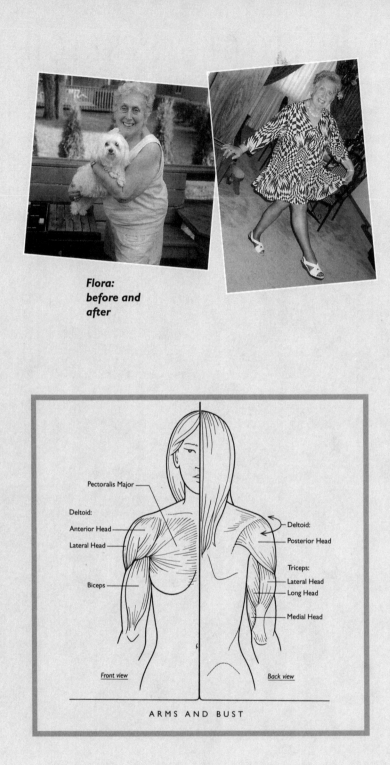

Flora:
before and
after

Pectoralis Major

Deltoid:

Anterior Head

Lateral Head

Biceps

Deltoid:

Posterior Head

Triceps:

Lateral Head

Long Head

Medial Head

Front view

Back view

ARMS AND BUST

UPPER BODY: ARMS, BUST, SHOULDERS AND UPPER BACK

Do you want to get rid of saggy arms and bra overhang? Do you want to develop and firm your chest muscles to achieve uplifted breasts and sexy shoulders? All it takes is a few of these upper body exercises to have a firmer, younger, more feminine figure, regardless of your age.

If you think lifting weights is for body builders, think again. Building muscle benefits anybody, at any age! Weight training is an integral part of my Hit the Spot Arms and Bust routine. It will improve your appearance, plus the best part of all is that it will improve your body's muscle-to-fat ratio, which will burn calories more efficiently, even as you sleep! Muscle is metabolically more active than fat, and thus it requires more calories to maintain. This will help you lose weight. My Hit the Spot Arms and Bust exercise plan zeros in on the arms, upper back, and shoulders and chest.

HOW OFTEN: I recommend you do at least four different upper body exercises three days a week . . . it will only take five minutes. To get the best contours, incorporate a variety into your routine: include an exercise for the upper back, one for the arms, one for the shoulders and one for the chest.

HOW MUCH WEIGHT: Dumbbells are great tools for training the upper body; they're convenient and effective and they let you work through a complete range of motion. To see results, you should do all these exercises with weights (except push-ups and tricep dips on chair). Begin using soup cans or three-pound hand weights (dumbbells). This is the quickest way to see true definition in the muscles.

- **If you can't perform six reps, you're probably trying to lift too much weight. Start with a lesser amount and work your way up!**

WHEN DO I INCREASE THE AMOUNT OF WEIGHT: When the last two reps feel too easy, it is time to move on to the next level of weights. Toning exercises should never be something you cruise through, but they should not be overwhelmingly painful either.

When you are able to complete all of the exercises in the program twice, with relative ease, it is time to think about increasing the intensity of the exercise. Gradual increases in weights are best. When doing reps, the last three should be pretty hard. Your muscles should be taxed by the last one. Suddenly adding a ten-pound dumbbell in each hand could injure you if you are not prepared for it. Go slowly. Start with soup cans if that is all you have. When you feel ready, purchase a set of hand-held weights. They are relatively inexpensive, but worth their weight in gold as far as results for you!

HOW MANY REPS? You should aim for one set of 8–12 reps of each exercise. As soon as you can complete this with relative ease, add a second set of 8–12 reps each exercise. I personally use five-pound weights in each hand and do two sets (16–24 reps). Rest 15 seconds between sets.

HIT THE SPOT TIP: If you are short on time, do one set (8–12 reps) with a heavier weight than you usually use to tax your muscle. Maximize your workout with a minimum of time.

BEAUTIFUL BACK

A well-developed back makes an incredible difference in your overall appearance. The development of your back determines the entire posture of your body, and a stronger back will keep your shoulders from slumping.

As you work out your back and it begins to take shape, you will notice that your waist will look smaller and so will your hips and buttocks. Because your back supports your shoulders, you will look better in all of your clothes!

ONE-ARM ROWS

I really love this exercise. Compared to a lot of the other exercises that I do, this one is easier, yet I find that it is one of the most effective things I can do for my back. Whenever I wear a strapless dress or a bathing suit, people tell me my back looks great. So guess what? I incorporate this exercise into almost all of my workouts!

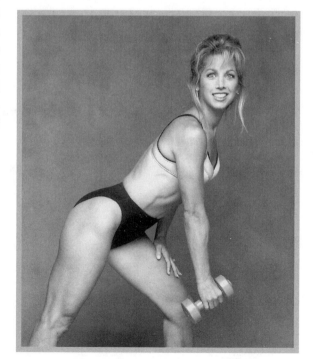

- **Stand with your feet apart as shown.**

- **Bend your knees slightly and keep your abs tight.**

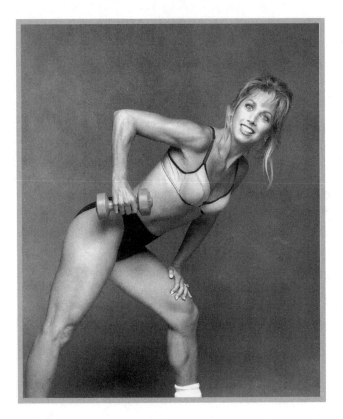

- Rest your palm on your front thigh or use a chair for support.

- Begin with your arm extended all the way down so you get a good stretch.

- Next, pull the weight up toward your armpit, and repeat.

- Watch your form.

- Be sure your back stays flat—don't round it.

BODY SHAPING . . . BODY SCULPTING . . .
NOT BODY BUILDING.

Upper-Back Firmer

- **Support knee and hand on chair.**

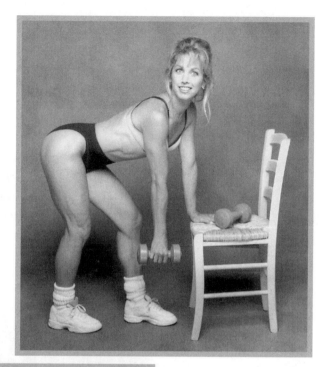

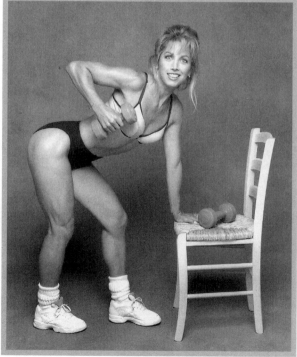

UPRIGHT ROWS

This is another great exercise for your back—and your shoulders, too! Unlike the previous back movement, this one focuses on the upper-middle part of the back. I assure you that if you start doing this exercise, people will take notice of your wonderfully developed back. In addition to making your back look great, this is also a great exercise for improving your posture!

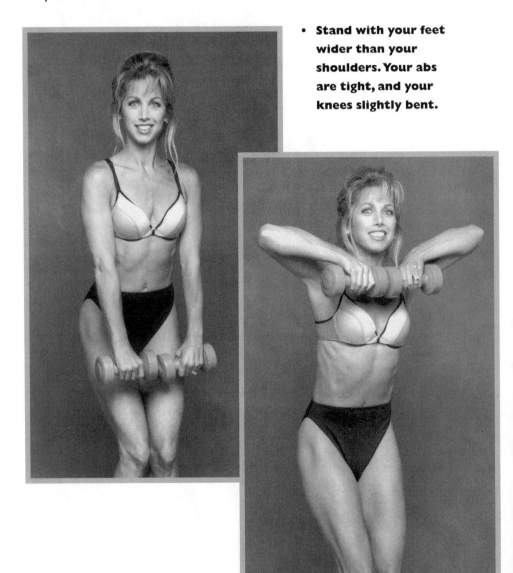

- **Stand with your feet wider than your shoulders. Your abs are tight, and your knees slightly bent.**

- **Hold the weights in your hands with your palms facing in.**

- **As you raise the weights, your arms should form the letter "V," as shown.**

- **Inhale as you lift. Squeeze your shoulder blades together, then return your arms to the starting position and exhale. Repeat.**

UPPER-BACK FIRMER

This is a great upper back exercise that targets "bra overhang." No more flab around your bra straps . . . This upper-back firmer is a difficult exercise, so just do the best you can. A few reps of this one really count!

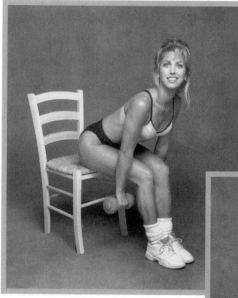

- **Sit on a chair with your legs out in front of you.**

- **Lean forward so that your chest is near your thighs.**

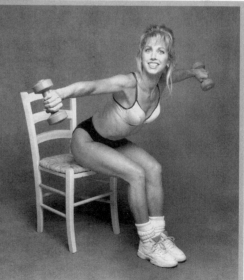

- **With the weights in your hands, slowly lift your arms straight out to the side, leading up with your pinkies.**

- **Squeeze your shoulder blades together. Return to starting position and repeat the movement.**

- **Make sure that your movement is slow and deliberate; try not to swing the weights.**

GREAT ARMS

You can wear baggy black pants to hide your hips, thighs and buttocks, but one of the most visible parts of your body are your arms. All of the upper-body exercises I have shown you also benefit your arms. However, it is important that you do some exercises specifically for your arms. I'm sure that we all had a teacher in elementary school who had flabby arms that would jiggle every time she wrote on the chalkboard. YUK! Granted, you'll have to do some cardio to get rid of the majority of the fat on your arms, but by doing these few simple exercises, you can make a huge difference in their look and shape.

BICEPS CURLS

This is a great exercise that can be done almost anywhere. I often do these one at a time while I'm talking on the phone or cooking dinner. Start with a weight that is pretty easy, maybe three or five pounds. If you don't have any hand weights, soup cans, small water bottles or your briefcase will work just fine. These can be done either together or alternating.

- **Stand with your feet wider than your hips. Your abs are tight, back is flat and knees are slightly bent.**

- **With an underhand grip, hold the weights at the front of your thighs.**

- **Exhale as you slowly raise the weights toward your upper arms and shoulders, bending your arms at the elbow.**

- Hold momentarily and return your hands to the starting position.

- Be sure that you keep your elbows close to your body throughout the movement.

- Watch your form.

- Make sure you don't arch your back when curling the weight.

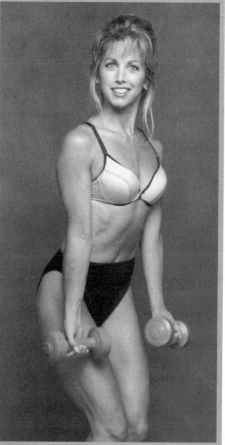

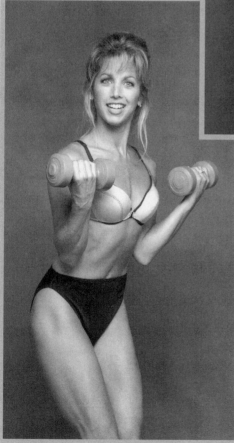

- Be sure not to swing the weights. Pause for a second at the bottom of the movement.

- Sit in a chair. Feel like your elbows are glued to your rib cage.

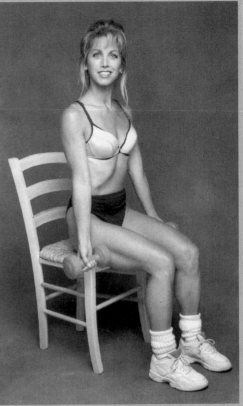

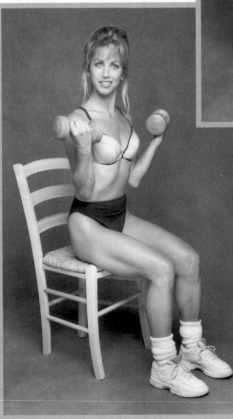

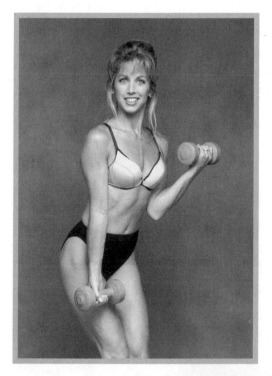

Alternating Bicep Curls

- **One at a time makes it easier.**

The Advanced Arm Curl
—*Intermediate*

- **One arm curls: double the weights and curl for one set, then switch arms.**

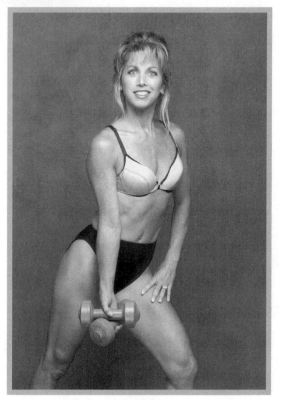

The Hammer Curl—*Advanced*

- **Instead of palms facing upward, face palms in and perform curls. Just turning your hands in targets a slightly different part of the biceps to show distinct definition in your arms.**

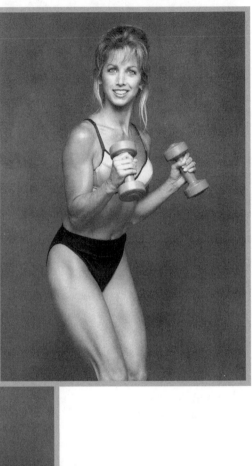

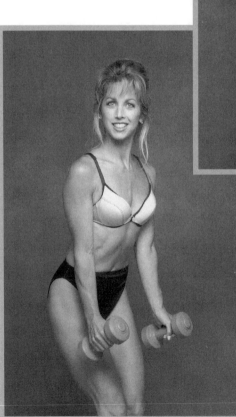

TRICEPS KICKBACK

Upper Body

No more underarm sag or underarm flab! We'll firm it up with these exercises designed to tone up the upper-back part of your arms and your triceps. Tightening these muscles will help you eliminate that jiggle on the back of your arms. Start with a comfortable weight, probably three or five pounds. You only need one hand weight to perform this exercise. This exercise should be done slowly. Don't let the weight swing like a pendulum.

- **Stand up with your left leg in front of your right and slightly bend the left knee.**

- **For support, rest your left hand on your left thigh.**

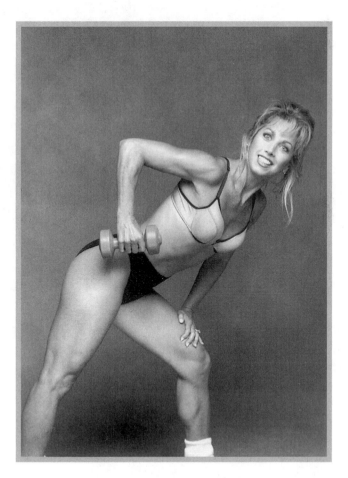

- **Keep your abs tight and your back flat.**

- **Raise your right elbow so that the upper part of your arm is parallel with the floor. Keep your elbow close to your body.**

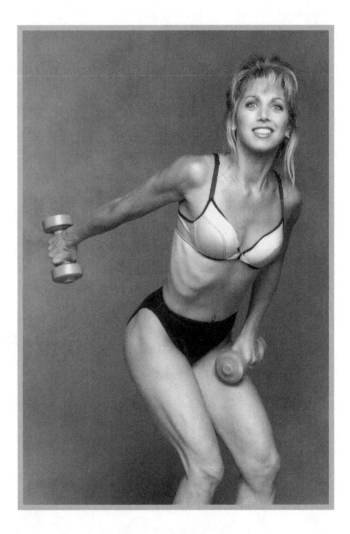

- **Straighten your right arm as shown. Be sure to squeeze your triceps as you straighten your arm.**

- **Return your right hand to the starting position, pause and repeat the movement.**

The Triceps Tightener

- **Hand supported on chair.**

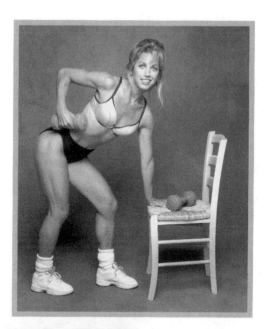

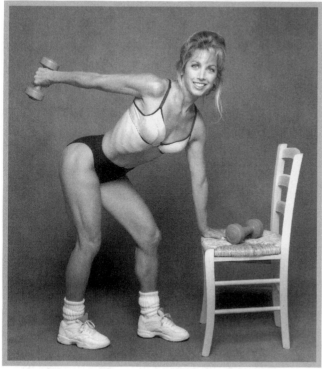

Double-Arm Lifts
— Advanced

- **Two-arm triceps kickback.**

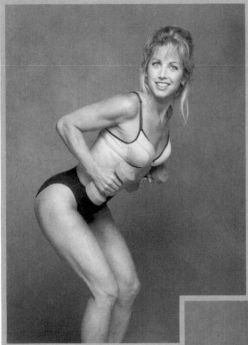

GET THOSE FIRM, SEXY ARMS YOU'VE ALWAYS WANTED.

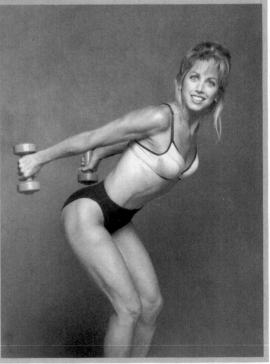

- **Double the weight to maximize your triceps workout.**

- **Hold both weights in one hand!**

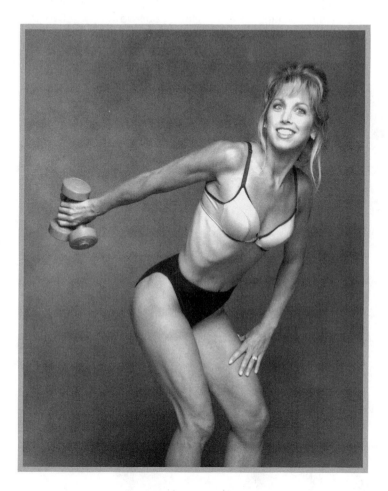

DECREASE YOUR REST PERIODS BETWEEN EXERCISES AS YOU GET STRONGER.

TRICEPS TONERS

Upper Body

Did you know that the triceps are one of the most underused muscles in the body? We always use our biceps (the front of the arms), carrying groceries or picking up our children, but we rarely get to use the backs of our arms. These exercises tone and strengthen the triceps in the back of the upper arm, so when we wave goodbye nothing jiggles. It is very important that you keep this movement under control. Simply slinging the weights around won't do you any good. Be careful not to hit yourself on the noggin, too! This exercise can be done either sitting or standing.

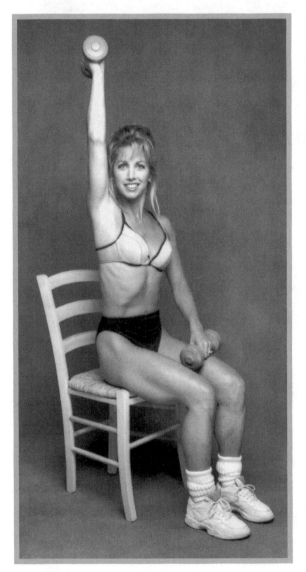

- **Sit in a chair, abs are tight and back straight.**

- **Hold the weight in your right hand and raise the weight over your head.**

- **Slowly bend your elbow and lower the weight behind your head as shown.**

- **Be sure to keep your elbow as close to your head as possible. We only want your triceps working during this one!**

- **Raise your hand back over your head to the starting position and squeeze your triceps as shown in photo.**

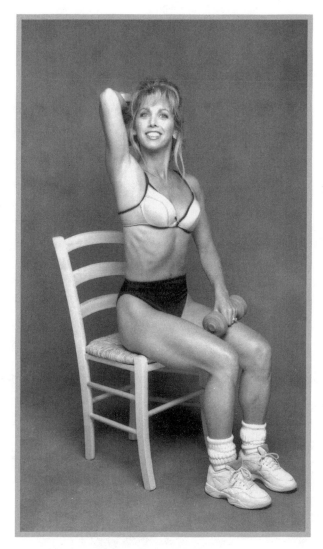

DRINK PLENTY OF WATER . . .
BEFORE, DURING, AND AFTER
YOUR WORKOUT!

Triceps Chair Dippers—*beginner*

- **Triceps dip on chair.**

- **Knees bent.**

- **Keep back straight, close to chair.**

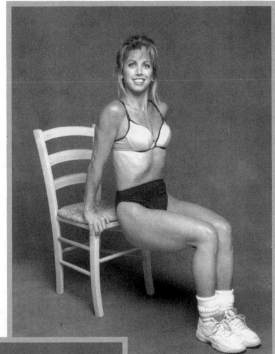

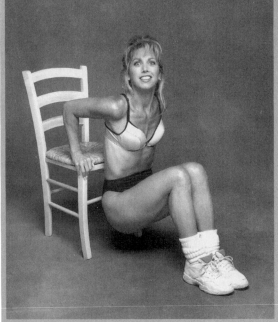

Triceps Dips—
advanced

- **Keep legs straight.**

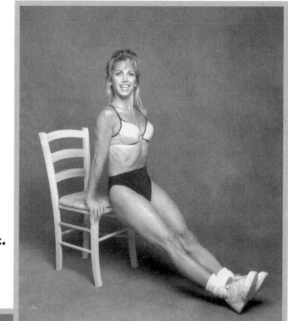

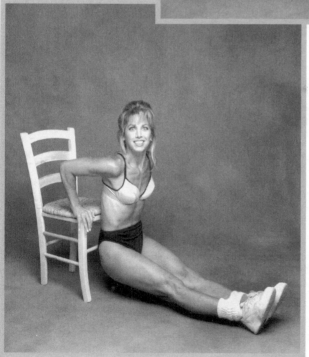

SEXY SHOULDERS

Weak and sloping shoulders can make you look tired. By developing these muscles you can create a wonderful appearance of youth, energy and self confidence.

Think about all the clothes that you own that have shoulder pads. Fortunately, by doing these exercises you won't have to depend on shoulder pads any longer! By developing strong, sexy shoulders, you will have that shapely look no matter what you wear.

You should aim for one set of 8–12 reps of each exercise. As soon as you can complete this with relative ease, add a second set of 8–12 reps of each exercise. Rest for 15 seconds between sets.

Let's try this quick lesson to understand exactly how your shoulder girdle moves and works. Try rounding your shoulders forward and then squeeze them back; next, lift them up toward your ears and then press them back down. There, you just exercised!

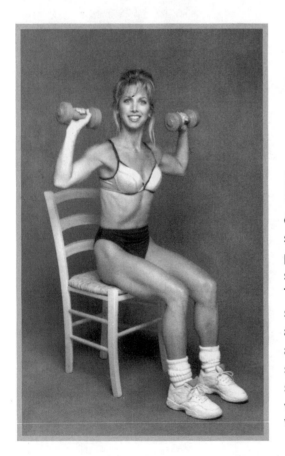

OVER-HEAD PRESSES

This is a great exercise for developing strong sexy muscles. So many people I meet have weak, sloping shoulders and poor posture. This will help! Throw your shoulder pads away; you aren't going to need them anymore. You are going to supply your own natural shoulder pads from now on with toned, firm muscles. With this exercise as well as the following two shoulder movements, start with 3–5 pound dumbbells. If they are too heavy, just do as many as you can and then finish the set with no weight at all until you build up some strength. With all exercises using weights, I want you to use a weight heavy enough so the last three or four repetitions are pretty challenging.

This exercise can also be done while sitting in a chair or standing, so do whichever is most comfortable.

- **Sit in a chair or stand with your feet shoulders' width apart, abs tight, back straight and knees slightly bent.**

- **Start with your hands at your shoulders.**

- **Exhale as you raise your hands over your head.**

- **Lower your arms to your shoulders and repeat.**

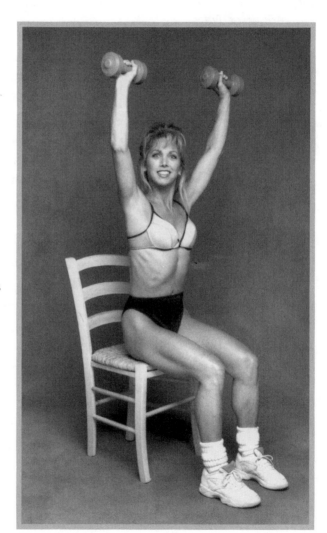

Rotator Cuff Strengthener

This exercise develops the muscles surrounding your shoulder joint. It's a great exercise to strengthen the shoulder girdle for any sports activities, especially tennis and golf. Also, if you find the next exercise (side raises) too hard, practice this one until your shoulder area becomes stronger. Try it . . . it's a small movement but very effective.

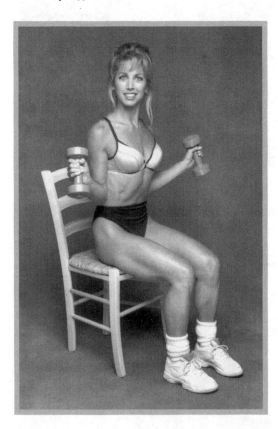

- **Sit or stand with elbows bent and held close to rib cage.**

- **Hold your forearms in front of your body.**

- **Open forearms out to sides, keeping elbows "glued" to rib cage.**

- **This is a small, controlled movement; keep your forearms parallel to the floor.**

SIDE RAISES

Upper Body

This one is a bit more difficult than the last shoulder exercise we did. (Can you imagine that?) This exercise really isolates the side of your shoulder. You will need to start this exercise with a smaller weight than the one you used for your overhead presses. Once you do them, I'm positive that you will feel exactly where it is targeting. It's very easy to get momentum going during this movement and lose the intent of the exercise. It should be done slowly and smoothly. You can sit in a chair for this one too!

- **Stand with your feet shoulders' width apart, abs tight, back straight and your knees slightly bent.**

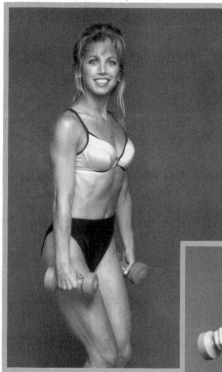

- **Start with your hands at your side as shown.**

- **This time I want you to inhale as you lift your hands up to just above your shoulders. Your arms should stay pretty straight during the movement although a slight bend in the elbow is okay.**

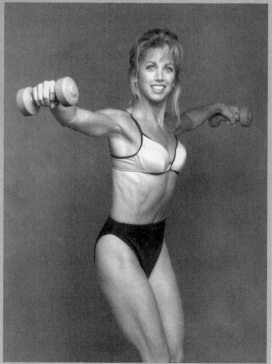

- **Now, slowly exhale, lowering your hands back to your sides. Repeat 8–12 times.**

FRONT RAISES

Upper Body

This exercise is almost identical to side raises, with one small change. You've got it—this time we raise the arms to the front. As with the side raises, be sure to concentrate on your form. I want you to keep the movement in your shoulders and not start swinging the weight around. Again, start with a light weight. If you find that it's too easy you can always add more later.

- **Stand with your feet shoulders' width apart, abs tight, back straight and your knees slightly bent.**

- **Start with your hands in front of you as shown.**

- **Inhale as you raise your arms (palms down) to just above your shoulders.**

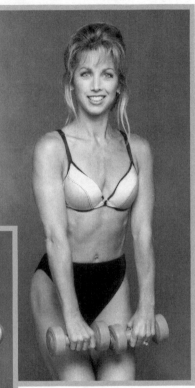

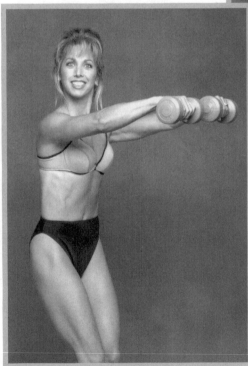

- **Slowly exhale and lower your arms to the starting position and repeat.**

Front Raises

- **Alternate front arm raises . . . they're a little easier to control.**

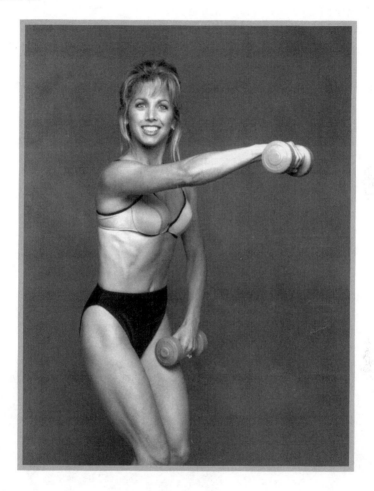

YOU ARE CREATING A BODY THAT IS STRONG AND BALANCED.

CHEST

Your chest is an important part of your body to exercise because it generally receives so much attention. The muscles of your chest (the pectorals) lift and give shape to your breasts, and a properly developed chest will enhance your firm and feminine figure.

When you work these muscles, you will develop an attractive line of cleavage, regardless of the size of your breasts. Furthermore, firm muscles underneath your breasts will help to counter the downward pull of gravity and help to form firm, uplifted breasts that might otherwise start to sag as time and age take their toll.

You should aim for one set of 8–12 repetitions of the exercises every time you do them. As soon as you can do this relatively easily, add a second set of 8–12 reps in each exercise. Rest 15 seconds between sets.

CHEST FIRMER (FLIES)

This is a great exercise for your chest. As you complete this movement, your arms should be bent as though you are hugging a beach ball. Make sure your lower back remains flat throughout the entire exercise. You can do this on the floor, on a step or on a bench for better range of motion.

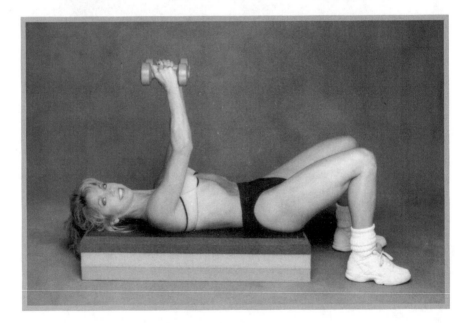

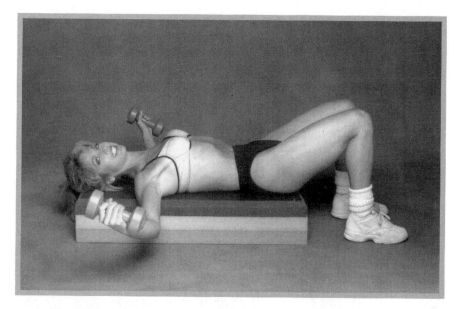

- **Lie on your back with your knees bent and your feet on the floor.**

- **Hold the weights in your hands with your arms extended at shoulder level, above your chest.**

- **Slowly lower your arms out to your side, keeping them bent at the same angle throughout the movement.**

- **Slowly return your arms to the starting position by *squeezing* your chest, and repeat the movement.**

CHEST PRESSES

This is another fabulous exercise designed to firm the muscles of your chest. Be sure that when you perform this movement, you keep your lower back pressed firmly into the floor, and avoid locking your elbows at the top of the movement. You can use a bench or step to really get a complete range of movement.

- **Lie on your back with your knees bent and your feet on the floor.**

- **With the weights in your hands, slowly bend your arms so that your elbows are parallel to your shoulders as shown.**

- **Push the weights straight up so that your arms are extended directly over your chest, as shown.**

- **Repeat the movement.**

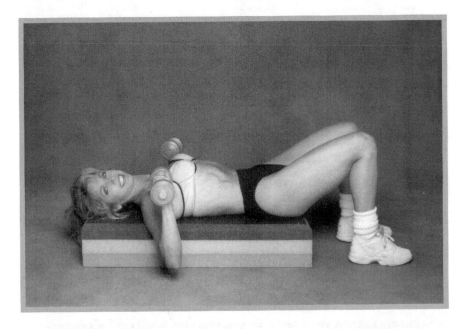

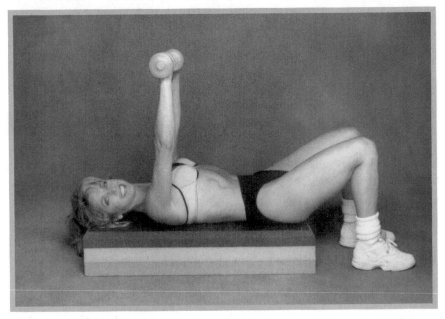

PUSH-UPS

A push-up is one of the best and most complete upper-body exercises. It's tried and true ... proven to work.

At first, this exercise should be done in a modified fashion. You can do this off your knees as soon as you develop enough upper-body strength to support your torso. Make sure that throughout the exercise you keep your back straight and your head slightly up. Bend your elbows and lower yourself as close to the floor as you can and still be able to return to the starting position. This is a very difficult exercise, so don't be discouraged if you are only able to do a couple. You'll get better at it. . . . I promise!

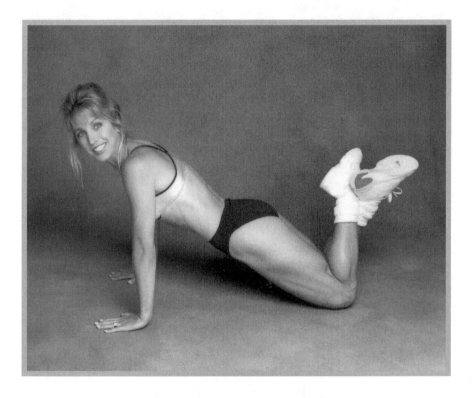

- **Kneel on a mat on the floor with your hands out in front of you.**

- **Straighten your back and keep your head in line with your spine.**

- **Slowly bend your elbows and lower your chest to the floor.**

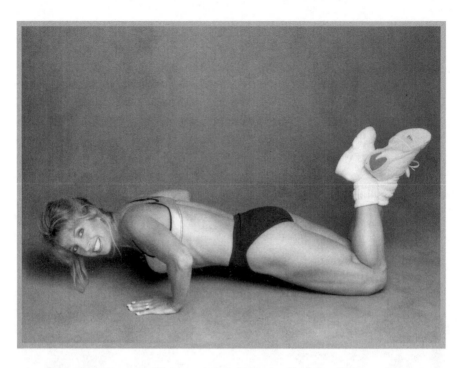

- **Straighten your elbows and return to the starting position.**

- **Repeat this movement as many times as you can.**

EXERCISE TO SLOW DOWN YOUR AGING PROCESS. FIFTY PERCENT OF AGING IS DUE TO AGE, BUT THE OTHER FIFTY PERCENT IS DUE TO THE UNDERUSE OF YOUR BODY. KEEP FIRM AND STAY YOUNG!

The Bench Push-Up

- **Try a push-up on a step or bench. . . . It might be easier for you.**

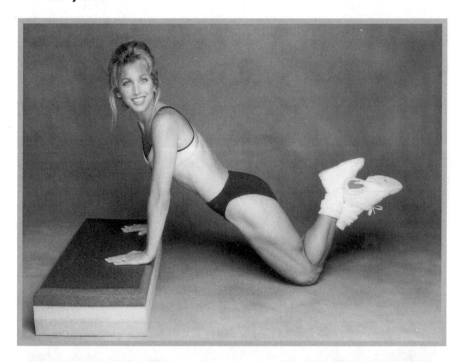

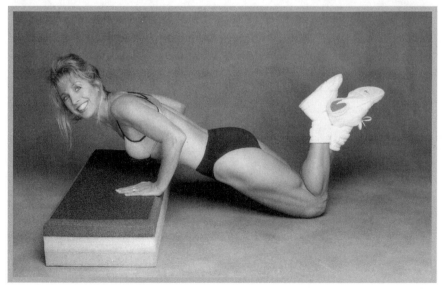

The Chest Developer—*Advanced*

- **Push-up on toes.**

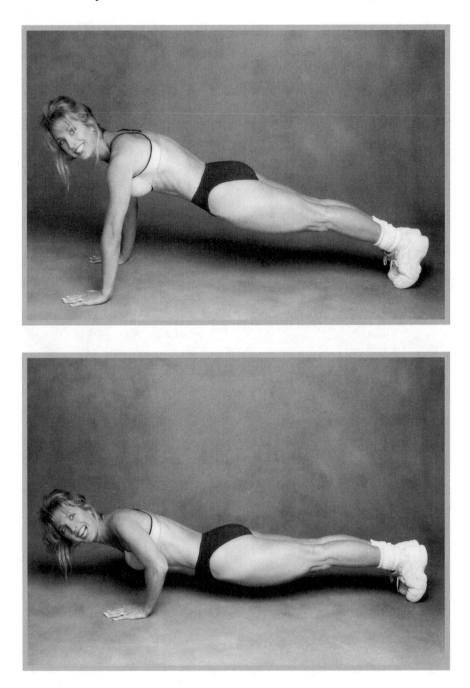

UPPER-BODY STRETCHES

Polish off the workout with a few stretches to elongate and lengthen the muscles! These are great to do after a weights workout, since the muscles have been contracted (shortened). (Hold each stretch 15–30 seconds.)

- **Triceps stretch.**

- **Give yourself a pat on the back for doing such a great job.**

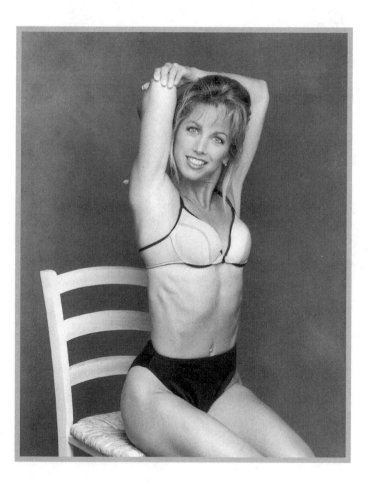

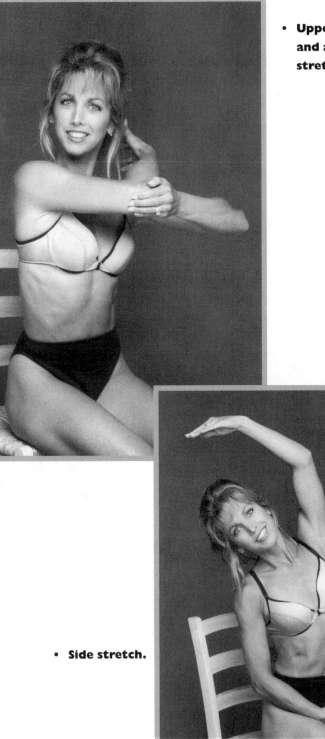

- **Upper back and arm stretch.**

- **Side stretch.**

TOTAL BODY MAKEOVER

On your way to losing inches, here are a few tips for things to do every day, because we need constant reminders if we are going to begin this change in lifestyle.

EACH DAY

- **Eat a good breakfast. (See daily samples on page 151.)**

- **Eat a nutritious lunch. (Choose from all the lunch options on pages 151.)**

- **Do some form of exercise for at least 10 minutes, either my Hit the Spot toning exercises or an aerobic activity such as walking.**

- **Think positive thoughts about yourself. . . or meditate for five minutes.**

- **Try to eat your dinner as early as possible.**

- **Brush your teeth after dinner to feel like you have finished eating for the night. This will prevent late-night snacking. . . the worst!**

EACH HOUR OF THE DAY

- **Drink water.**

- **Take three deep breaths.**

- **Think good posture . . . pull in your tummy and tighten your abs.**

PICK THE SHAPE
YOU WANT TO
BE IN FROM
THREE FITNESS
CATEGORIES

1. To be healthy and lose up to one pound per week, exercise three times per week with a 30-minute aerobic workout and two times per week with my 10-minute Hit the Spot (muscle-toning) workout.

2. To look great in clothes and lose up to two pounds per week, exercise four times per week with a 30-minute aerobic workout and three times per week with my 10-minute Hit the Spot (muscle-toning) workout.

3. To be in perfect bikini shape, exercise five times per week with a 30-minute aerobic workout and three times per week with my 30-minute Hit the Spot (muscle-toning) workout.

And, of course, eat well . . . and follow my Hit the Spot Pyramid Diet Plan!

WEEK I WORKOUT

AEROBIC / CARDIO WORKOUTS: see options on page 132

20-minute walk, three times a week

MUSCLE TONING

Hit the Spot: 10-Minute Workout, three times a week

	EXERCISE	PAGE #	SPOT TONING ZONE
1	WIDE-STANCE SQUAT OR BUN LUNGE	52	HIPS AND BUNS ZONE
2	GREAT GLUTES SQUAT	84	
3	BICEPS	98	ARMS, BUST AND SHOULDER ZONE
4	TRICEPS TONERS	108	
5	OVERHEAD PRESSES	112	
6	CHEST FIRMER	118	
7	LOWER-TUMMY TIGHTENER	32	AB ZONE
8	CRUNCH	27	
9	OUTER-THIGH TRIMMER	53	THIGH ZONE
10	INNER-THIGH FIRMER	57	
	FLEXIBILITY		
1	QUAD STRETCH	73	
2	BUTTOCKS STRETCH	89	

*Perform 8-10 repetitions of each exercise going through them in the order that I have shown. Go through the list TWICE. It would be best to do this routine three days a week with at least one day of rest between each muscle-toning workout. Make sure that you do your stretches at the **end** of your workout.*

WEEK 2 WORKOUT

AEROBIC / CARDIO WORKOUT: see page 132

25-minute walk, three times a week

MUSCLE TONING

Hit the Spot: 10-Minute Workout, three times a week

	EXERCISE	PAGE #	SPOT TONING ZONE
1	LUNGE DIPS WITH CHAIR	49	HIPS AND THIGHS ZONE
2	ONE-ARM ROWS	93	ARMS, BUST AND SHOULDER ZONE
3	UPRIGHT ROWS	96	
4	CHEST PRESS	119	
5	LEVEL 2 CRUNCH	28	AB ZONE
6	WAISTLINE SLIMMERS	37	
7	BICYCLES	38	
8	BOTTOMS UP	76	BUNS ZONE
9	TUSH TIGHTENER	78	
10	BUTT TAPS	82	
	FLEXIBILITY		
1	HIP AND THIGH STRETCH	73	
2	UPPER BACK AND ARM STRETCH	126	

This week attempt 8-12 reps of each exercise. Complete in this order twice!

WEEK 3 WORKOUT

AEROBIC / CARDIO WORKOUTS: see options on page 132

25-minute walk, three times a week

MUSCLE TONING

Hit the Spot: 10-Minute Workout, three times a week

	EXERCISE	PAGE #	SPOT TONING ZONE
1	POWER LUNGE	49	LEGS AND BUNS ZONE
2	SQUATS	50	
3	HAMSTRING CURLS	62	
4	UPPER-BACK FIRMER	97	ARMS, BUST AND UPPER-BACK ZONE
5	BICEPS CURL	98	
6	SIDE RAISES	114	
7	FRONT RAISES	116	
8	THE ROPE-CLIMB CRUNCH	30	AB ZONE
9	LOWER-TUMMY TIGHTENER	34	
10	WAISTLINE TRIMMER	36	
	FLEXIBILITY		
1	HAMSTRING STRETCH	142	
2	SIDE STRETCH	126	

This is your third week. Let's step it up a little. I want you to do 16-24 repetitions of each exercise. Try to add weights when possible.

AEROBIC/CARDIO OPTIONS

WALKING

STAIR CLIMBING (ON A MACHINE OR STAIRS AT HOME)

JOGGING

RUNNING

HIKING

SWIMMING

BIKE RIDING (STATIONARY BIKE)

ROWING MACHINE

STEP AEROBICS

WATER AEROBICS

AEROBICS (LOW- OR HIGH-IMPACT AEROBICS)

AEROBIC RIDERS

DANCING

CROSS-COUNTRY SKIING OR CROSS-COUNTRY SKIING MACHINES

ICE SKATING

GLIDE SLIDE (SLIDE BOARD)

ROLLER SKATING/ROLLER BLADING/IN-LINE SKATING

JUMP ROPE

REBOUNDING/MINI TRAMPOLINE

TIPS FOR SUCCESS

- **Work at least 12 minutes; go for 30 minutes.**

- **Try varying the activities to stay motivated.**

- **Cross-train to work different muscle groups—for instance, I like to do a fast walk on Monday, step aerobics on Wednesday, and my aerobic rider or cycling on Friday.**

HIT THE SPOT WEEKLY EXERCISE DIARY

- **Check each box if you've completed at least 5 minutes of a specific zone (body spot).**

- **In each aerobics box note the type of aerobic exercise you completed, such as walking, cycling, step aerobics, and so on, and then note the time and distance.**

Hit the Spot Weekly Exercise Diary

ZONE	Day 1	Day 2	Day 3	Day 4	Day 5	Day 6	Day 7
ABS							
BUNS							
HIPS AND THIGHS							
ARMS AND BUST							
AEROBIC							

Fill out:

Number of days you did aerobics this week _____

Weekly total hours/minutes _____

Number of days you "Hit the Spot" _____

Weekly total hours/minutes _____

HERE'S A COMPLETE PLAN FOR YOU: YOU WOULDN'T BUILD A HOUSE WITHOUT A BLUEPRINT—START NOW!

REMEMBER: MUSCLE-TONING EXERCISING IS TRULY THE SECRET TO BURNING THE MAXIMUM FAT DAY AND NIGHT!

A HEALTHY BACK

Almost 80 percent of all Americans will, at some point in their lives, suffer from debilitating back pain. In fact, estimates indicate that approximately six-and-one-half million people are incapacitated on any given day. The United States Health Service estimates that back problems are the most frequent cause of activity limitation in Americans under the age of 40, as well as the third most prevalent disabling condition in over-40 Americans. Back pain, however, is often preventable. Your spine is your life: keep it strong!

Back pain is a debilitating disorder that reflects our living habits. The majority of back pain is a muscular response to overload. Realizing and understanding the causes of back pain will put you in control and allow *you* to help your back. Although experts theorize that 80 percent of back problems are degenerative in nature, stemming from misuse (poor lifting technique) or lack of use, a number of other factors can also contribute to back pain.

- **WEAK ABDOMINAL MUSCLES**—Weak abdominal muscles are the result of improper exercise. Without strong tummy muscles, the muscles of your lower back have to work double duty to keep your body upright.

- **TIGHT HAMSTRING MUSCLES**—Tight hamstrings (the muscles in the back of the thighs) can trigger back pain by pulling on the pelvis, which in turn pulls on the lower spine.

- **WEAK BACK MUSCLES**—Muscles not exercised will deteriorate; therefore, weak and unexercised back muscles will provide inferior support of the spine.

- **EMOTIONAL STRESS/CHRONIC FATIGUE**—Many experts believe that stress is the single most important causal factor contributing to back pain. The spinal musculature is overstressed by chronic emotional fatigue. Relaxation techniques and proper coping mechanisms can be implemented when fatigue is the cause of back pain.

- **OVERWEIGHT**—Poor nutrition and lack of exercise contribute to excessive abdominal weight. The more weight you have in your stomach, the more stress is put on your back.

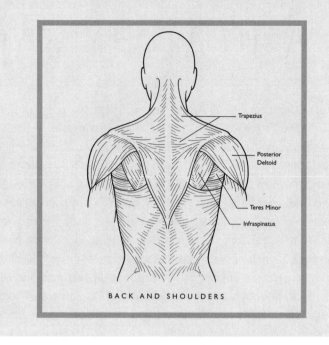

BACK AND SHOULDERS

Labels on image: Trapezius, Posterior Deltoid, Teres Minor, Infraspinatus

SPECIAL BACK STRENGTHENERS

Here is a personal back-care program that will help prevent future problems. The following exercises are for anyone who has suffered from back problems, as well as for everyone who wants to prevent back problems from ever becoming a part of their lives! Always begin the exercises with a warm-up.

WARM-UP: Begin with a five-minute warm-up: brisk walking, stationary cycling or just marching in place.

NOTE: If you are in pain right now, do not do these exercises until your back pain has subsided. Rest is best at first, then gradually begin this rehabilitation and prevention routine *after* you have checked with your doctor.

IT'S TIME TO GET STARTED . . . NOW!

PELVIC TILT

This exercise stretches your back and strengthens your abdominal muscles, which relieves pressure on your lower back and thus helps prevent swayback. Plus, it's great for the lower tummy.

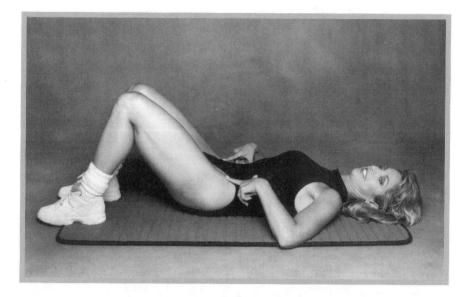

- Lie on your back on the floor with your knees bent and feet flat (place a towel underneath your buttocks—optional).

- Rotate your pelvis up so your back flattens against the floor and the front of your hips (hip bones) moves closer to your rib cage.

- Contract your abs, exhale and hold the position for 3–5 seconds.

- Repeat this movement 8–12 times.

HALF SIT-UPS

This exercise is an excellent way to strengthen the muscles of the abdominal and lower back regions. Make sure you keep your lower back flat throughout the movement.

- **Lie on your back on the floor with your knees bent.**

- **Place your arms in front of your chest.**

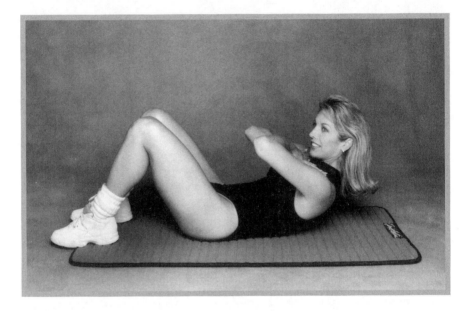

- **Contract and exhale as you slowly lift your head and shoulders about 6 inches from the floor.**

- **Hold the position for 3–5 seconds.**

- **Slowly return to starting position.**

- **Repeat this movement 8–12 times.**

ELBOW PROPS

Do this exercise to help maintain the normal lumbar curve and to strengthen the muscles of the lower back. Make sure your hips stay flat on the floor.

- **Lie on your stomach on the floor.**

- **Place your arms at your sides, hands palm down next to your shoulders.**

- **Prop yourself up on your elbows while pressing your hips to the floor and squeeze your buttocks. Hold this position for 15–20 seconds.**

- **Return to starting position and relax. Repeat twice.**

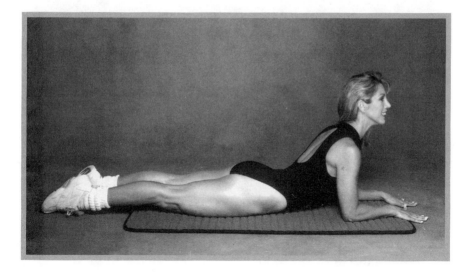

OPPOSITE ARM/LEG LIFTS

Do this exercise to strengthen the buttocks, lower-back muscles and specifically the back extensors (the middle and upper back muscles). Make sure that when you lift your leg, your hips and pelvis stay pressed firmly to the floor.

- **Lie face down on the floor with a towel under your chin for comfort.**

- **Extend your arms overhead, hands palm down.**

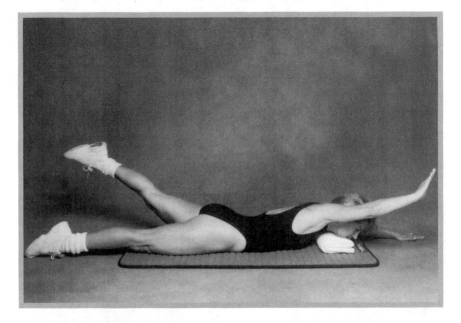

- **Make sure that your head stays in line with your spine (nose pointed to the floor).**

- **Raise your right arm and your left leg at the same time. Hold lift for 4 counts.**

- **Return to starting position and repeat with opposite arm and leg.**

- **Repeat this movement 3 times, alternating sides each time.**

BACK RELAXER

This exercise increases back flexibility, reduces pressure on your back (especially from fatigue and emotional tension) and cools you down.

- **Lie on your back, bend your knees to your chest and bear hug, grasping hands under thighs.**

- **Press the small of the back against the floor, keep abdomen flat and pretend that the navel is pressing into your spine.**

- **Hold for 15–20 seconds, breathing deeply.**

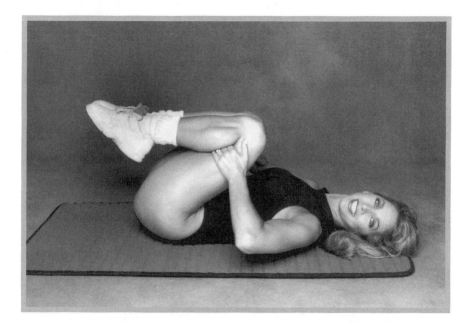

HAMSTRING STRETCH

Back

This is a great stretch that isolates the hamstrings. It's important to keep your hamstrings flexible and supple to allow the lower back to relax and be in perfect alignment. For those of you with tight hamstrings, a towel will help you to feel the stretch.

- **Lie on your back on the floor, with your knees bent and your feet on the floor.**

- **Raise your right leg up and grasp it with both hands.**

- **Straighten your right leg and raise it toward your chest.**

- **Hold the stretch for 15–20 seconds.**

- **Lower the leg to the floor and repeat the stretch on the left leg.**

HIT THE SPOT
MINI IMPROVERS

Hit the Spot: Mini Chin Lift

A flabby double chin is caused by sagging, unused muscle. You can tighten those muscles under the chin to tone and firm up the three muscle groups that directly affect your double chin and have a more youthful, trimmer profile. Do this exercise daily as you read or watch TV It only takes a few seconds to ward off that double chin!

Open your mouth. Bite upward with the lower jawline and your lower teeth, feeling it under the chin. Hold for five seconds.

Hit the Spot: Neck Relaxer

I put in 150,000 miles aloft every year. To ward off flying fatigue—poor circulation from all that sitting builds up kinks and tension in the neck—I've devised a neck relaxer that I can do in my seat. My seat companion, seeing what I'm doing, often joins in. (Tip: Drink one glass of water every hour you are in the air—it prevents dehydration and jet lag.)

Sit up straight, with your shoulders relaxed, your neck extended nice and tall. Lower your left ear slowly to your left shoulder. Hold for 15 seconds. Roll your head to the right and hold your right ear to your right shoulder for 15 seconds.

Roll your head to the center. Touch your chin to your chest for 15 seconds. Keeping your chin to your chest, rock your head slowly to the left, then to the right. Semicircle continuously for 15 seconds. Be sure to keep your neck long throughout the entire exercise.

Relax. Never jerk your head or roll it backward or in a full circle—such movements can compress the top two vertebrae and cause injury.

BENEFITS: Keeps your neck from getting stiff, relaxes stiff neck and aching head.

Hit the Spot: Jaw Relaxer

Does your jaw feel tense most of the time? Do you grind your teeth when you sleep, or do you clench your jaw when you are under pressure? Do you get headaches at or near your temples along with pain at the sides of your neck? If the symptoms sound familiar, you just might have *temporomandibular joint syndrome*. (It is more commonly called T.M.J., and it afflicts tens of millions of Americans.) Check with your doctor or your dentist, especially if your jaw makes clicking, popping or grating noises.

Some of us have habits that simply cause tension in the jaw. We clench a pencil between our lips or teeth, cradle a telephone between neck and shoulder, chew gum constantly or bite our fingernails, all of which can cause excess tension in the jaw.

If you do suffer from T.M.J., this might help. One way is to learn to relax your jaw whenever you are not eating or talking.

Press the tip of your tongue against the roof of your mouth. Hold this position for 15 seconds.

Relax for 15 seconds.

Open your mouth as wide as possible.

Place three fingers, stacked vertically, between your teeth. (If your jaw muscles are so tight that three fingers will not fit, try two.) Hold for 15 seconds.

BENEFITS: If you do this exercise regularly, within a couple of weeks you will notice reduced tension and pain in the jaw.

Hit the Spot: Minifacial

Why do you think they are called *worry wrinkles?* It is because wrinkles set in when you are thinking about a problem and your face becomes tense. It takes more muscles to frown than to smile. When your face is set in a worried expression, wrinkles start spreading like ripples on a pond. I have discovered a quick massage that gives your face a break from all of that.

Place your index fingers at the inside corners of your eyes, on either side of the bridge of your nose. Make small circles on your skin. Keep making small circles as you work your index fingers all the way around your eyes.

Rub the bridge of your nose. Work up and across your eyebrows.

Make three small circles over each temple. Make three circles from the middle of your forehead out and up toward your hairline.

Repeat twice.

Massage your cheeks and jaw with your thumbs and the pads of your fingertips—gently, gently.

Rub small sections of skin with light, quick motions, starting at the chin and moving up and out along the cheeks and jaw, for a count of 10.

BENEFITS: Releases tension, improves complexion by increasing circulation to your skin, feels fantastic. Who could ask for anything more?

Hit the Spot: Shoulder Relaxer

A few hours of inactivity can make your shoulders ache. Tension collects behind your neck, and at the points your arms join the trunk of your body you can fell like Atlas carrying the world on your shoulders. The best relief is an exercise that decreases muscle tension. Lift your shoulders to your ears. Inhale. Lower your shoulders and exhale.
Repeat.

Roll your shoulders up and back 5 times.
Roll your shoulders up and forward 5 times.

BENEFITS: Releases tension and reduces stiffness in your neck and shoulders.

Hit the Spot: No More Slouching

Perfect posture says a lot about a person. Body-language studies reveal that people who sit up straight project authority and confidence. This stretch will improve your posture and help you project such an image.

Clasp your fingers behind your neck.
Pull your elbows back as far as you can. Hold for 5 seconds.
Keeping your fingers clasped, try to bring your elbows to touch together in front of you. Hold for 5 seconds.
Release your hands and relax for 5 seconds.
Repeat the sequence twice.

BENEFITS: Keeps you from slouching, stretches your pecs, eases you into a positive posture.

Hit the Spot: Foot Massage

Your poor, aching feet! Think about them for a while. You walk on them all the time. You stuff them into shoes that are too tight. You stub them, you get them wet. They get no respect. When was the last time you soaked them in warm, sudsy water? Maybe, just maybe, you rub them at night, but that is not enough. Feet need massaging before they reach the point of exhaustion. All you need is a minute—let's say while you are watching TV—and a tennis ball.

Take off your shoes and socks.
Place a tennis ball under one foot.
Roll the ball back and forth under the foot for 30 seconds.
Switch feet and repeat.

BENEFITS: Loosens up your feet—your whole body will follow suit.

Hit the Spot: Writer's Cramp Reliever

After hearing friends complain about writer's cramp, I discovered it firsthand when I began writing *JumpStart* and this book. Writer's cramp is the tensing of muscles in the fingers and in the hand joints. It usually is caused by gripping a pencil or pen too tightly. Hackers get cramps in their figures and hands, too. I designed this exercise to relieve and prevent stress buildup in the hands. Ward off writer's cramp by doing this flex before you start on the computer or put pen to paper.

Stand or sit up straight.

Extend your right arm (or left, if you are left-handed) straight out in front of your body, palm up. With the opposite hand, grasp the fingers of the extended hand and bend them back as far as you can without causing pain.

Hold for 15 seconds.

Release.

Turn the palm of your extended arm, grasp the fingers with the opposite hand and bend them toward the palm. Hold for 15 seconds.

Repeat.

B E N E F I T S : **Releases tension in your hands, wrists, fingers and forearms.**

ASK DENISE

WHAT IS THE BEST TIME OF THE DAY TO EXERCISE?

Toning can be done anytime. . . . that's the best part of my Hit the Spot exercise program! You can do five minutes here, you can do five minutes there—in the morning, afternoon and/or evening—whenever you can squeeze in the time! So even the busiest person can find time to Hit the Spot!

DOES ONLY 10 MINUTES OF EXERCISE REALLY WORK?

It sure does! Toning exercises are a great way to isolate and strengthen a muscle—with each repetition you are firming that area. With only 10 minutes a day you can target and tone your abs, hips and thighs, arms and bust! The best part about my program is that you don't have to take a chunk of time out of your busy schedule. You can divide my 10-minute Hit the Spot exercises throughout the day!

You get the same benefit if you break it up into 10-minute routines, whereas with aerobics you need 20–30 consecutive minutes.

HOW MANY DAYS A WEEK SHOULD I EXERCISE AEROBICALLY?

Three to four days per week is ideal for burning fat, increasing your aerobic capacity and really reshaping your body. That is not to say that if you can only fit it in twice a week you will not get anything out of it. . . . you will! But there is no doubt that the more often you exercise aerobically, the faster you will lose fat and achieve the results you are looking for.

WHAT IF I HAVE NO TIME TO EXERCISE?

One of the most basic principles of my philosophy of fitness is that everyone can find time to exercise, even if they have to squeeze it in among their daily chores. Some of my favorite recommendations to someone with a hectic schedule are: walk or bike to work or to the train station instead of driving; keep a set of light hand weights at the office for quick upper-body toning or park in the last spot in the parking lot and walk the rest of the way! All exercise adds up. Look for ways to exercise creatively as a part of your busy day. Turn that idle time into toning time.

SHOULDN'T I LOSE WEIGHT BEFORE I START TO LIFT WEIGHTS?

No. This is a common misconception. A lot of people think that if they have fat on their body and they start to lift weights, their fat will turn into muscle. This is impossible. Fat is fat and muscle is muscle! They are not interchangeable or components of each other. In fact, lifting weights actually contributes to fat loss, since the added muscle increases your metabolism. And speeding up that metabolism helps you to lose weight even more quickly.

WHAT IS THE BEST WAY TO SPEED UP MY METABOLISM?

The top three components to speeding your metabolism are:

1. **Never skip a meal. It will slow down your metabolism. Eat several times a day. Don't give your metabolism a chance to rest! Follow my Hit the Spot pyramid plan—it will keep your metabolism up and the pounds down!**

2. **Add toning exercises like my Hit the Spot program to your routine. Remember, the more you increase your muscle tone, the more fat you burn!**

3. **Exercise aerobically at a low intensity for 20 minutes three days a week. It does wonders for fat loss!**

WALKING AEROBIC?

Yes! Aerobic walking burns fat! To be aerobic, by definition, you must elevate your heart rate. I walk 120 steps per minute—that is equal to a 15-minute–mile walk. For a starter pace, try to walk about an 18-minute–mile walk. One of the reasons that my TrimWalk tape has been so successful is that I keep pace for you! So, put some spring in that step and let your arms move and pump with you, whether you are enjoying nature's bounty or on a treadmill watching your favorite TV show. You can walk your way to a better body!

HIT THE SPOT PYRAMID DIET

The Food Guide Pyramid is everywhere! It's on your bread bag, your milk carton and in your kids' schoolbooks. The pyramid is all around you because it's an easy way to think about healthful eating. (See page 162.) It's as simple as this: Eat more foods from the bigger boxes at the bottom (grains, fruits and vegetables), and less food from the smaller boxes at the top (oils, fats and sweets).

But "eat more" and "eat less" aren't helpful unless you can get a handle on what's right for you, so I've designed three eating plans based on the Food Guide Pyramid.

The 1350 calorie plan is about right for sedentary women and older adults who are trying to lose weight. The 1600 calorie plan will keep those folks at their current weight, but will create gradual, healthy, weight loss for active women and sedentary men. The 2200 calorie plan will produce gradual weight loss for active men and some very active women.

But you won't have to count calories or fat grams! Because each daily sample plan is between 20 and 25 percent fat.

Choose the category that's right for you, then check this Daily Exchange Chart. You'll find the food group servings you need daily to build a healthy body. When you use the Food Guide Pyramid to build your Hit the Spot diet you'll get all the protein, vitamins and minerals you need for maximum energy and healthy weight loss.

Daily Exchange Totals

	1350	1600	2200
Dairy	2	2	2
Fruit	2	3	4
Vegetables	3	4	5
Grain	6	6	9
Starch	1	2	3
Protein	2	2	2
Fat	4	6	8
Crave Stopper	1	1	1

To make healthy eating easier for you, I've divided the pyramid food groups into a suggested plan for three meals and a snack each day. You can arrange them differently if another pattern suits your lifestyle better. Notice that in my plan, I've arranged the meals so you're getting most of your food during the day, when you're most active, and need more fuel from food. That means you won't be starving all day long (which causes bingeing later on). You'll think more clearly, feel more energetic and better coordinated all day long, and feel more in control when dinner time rolls around. Dinner is a light meal, because, if you're like most people, you'll need less energy in the evening.

Sample Plan

	1350	1600	2200
BREAKFAST			
Dairy	1	1	1
Fruit	1	1	1
Grain	3	4	5
Fat	0	2	2
LUNCH			
Dairy	1	1	1
Fruit	1	1	1
Vegetable	1	2	2
Grain	2	2	4
Protein	1	1	1
Fat	2	2	2
SNACK			
Crave Stopper	1	1	1
Fruit	1	1	1
DINNER			
Fruit	1	1	1
Vegetable	2	2	3
Grain	1	0	0
Starch	1	2	3
Protein	1	1	1
Fat	2	2	4

Hit the Spot Weekly Food Plan "At a Glance"

ZONE	Day 1	Day 2	Day 3	Day 4	Day 5	Day 6	Day 7
BREAKFAST	Cereal	Breakfast sandwich	Yogurt/ Cereal	Graham crackers and peanut butter	Bagel and cheese	Oatmeal	Waffles
LUNCH	Ham and cheese sandwich	Roast beef sandwich	Turkey and cheese pita	Grilled chicken salad	Egg salad sandwich	Hot dog and slaw	Tuna salad sandwich
SNACK	Chocolate pudding and banana	Juice and cookies	Fat free potato chips and juice	Fat free ice cream and fruit	Lowfat popcorn and juice	Cookies and juice	Yogurt and fruit
DINNER	Oriental stir fry	Grilled tuna steaks	Tortilla scramble	Pasta Italiano	Poached salmon	Dijon chicken	Grilled pork tenderloin

Hit the Spot Weekly Food Diary

ZONE	Day 1	Day 2	Day 3	Day 4	Day 5	Day 6	Day 7
DAIRY (2)							
FRUIT (2-4)							
VEGETABLES (3-5)							
GRAIN (6-9)							
STARCH (1-3)							
PROTEIN (2)							
FAT (4-8)							
CRAVE STOPPER (1)							

- **Check each box when you've eaten each type of food.**

- **You might mark more than one box for a food. For exam-
  ple, a little piece of chicken wil count as one protein and
  one fat.**

_____ Number of days you ate well.

_____ Number of days you drank at least 8 glasses of water.

_____ Average number of hours slept nightly.

What are your goals for the next week?

_____

HOW MUCH IS
A SERVING?

Of course you'll need to know how much food is in each serving, so take a look at each group, and find your favorite foods. Just plug them into the calorie-level plan that's right for you, and you'll have satisfying menus that meet your needs, and keep your weight under control.

LEAN PROTEIN EXCHANGES

(70 calories, 14 gm protein, 0 carbohydrate, 2 gm fat)
Despite the fact that these protein portions are small, they still add up to the high-protein diet you need to maintain muscle while you lose weight. The secret? You also get protein from dairy foods, grains, starches and vegetables. Eating Food Guide Pyramid-style with small servings of lean meat, chicken, fish, beans and eggs and larger servings from the bottom of the pyramid pro-vides all the nutrition you need to build a healthy body.

COUNT AS ONE PROTEIN

Chicken or turkey white meat, no skin . . . . 2 oz.

Fish: cod, flounder, haddock, halibut, trout,
          tuna (fresh or canned in water). . . . . 2 oz.

Shellfish: clams, crab, lobster, oysters, scallops,
    shrimp, surimi (imitation shellfish) . . . . 2 oz.

Cheese: fat-free or 1% cottage cheese . . . . 1/2 cup

    fat-free cheese. . . . . 2 oz.

Eggs: whole 1

    whites 4

    egg substitute. . . . . 1/2 cup

Deli meats: hot dog, sausage, sliced meats
    (1 gram fat per ounce) . . . . 2 oz.

COUNT AS ONE PROTEIN PLUS ONE FAT

Lean beef: round, sirloin, flank, tenderloin,
    rump, porterhouse steak, ground
    round (fat trimmed) . . . . 2 oz.

Lean pork: fresh ham, boiled ham, Canadian
    bacon, tenderloin, center loin chops
    (fat trimmed). . . . . 2 oz.

Lamb or veal chops: fat trimmed . . . . 2 oz.

Chicken or turkey: dark meat, white meat
    with skin . . . . 2 oz.

Fish: salmon, catfish, bluefish, sardines,
    drained oil-packed tuna. . . . . 2 oz.

Cheese: 4.5% cottage cheese . . . . 1/2 cup

    grated parmesan . . . . 1/4 cup

    process cheese (3 grams fat or less per ounce) . . . . 2 oz.

Deli meats: hot dog, sausage, sandwich meats
    (less than 3 grams fat per ounce) . . . . 2 oz.

DAIRY EXCHANGES

**(90 to 100 calories, 8 gm protein, 12 gm
carbohydrate, up to 3 grams fat)**

COUNT AS ONE DAIRY EXCHANGE:

Milk: skim, 1%, lowfat buttermilk . . . . 1 cup

Evaporated skim milk . . . . 1/2 cup

Nonfat dry milk (dry, before mixing) . . . . 1/3 cup

Yogurt: nonfat plain or nonfat
       artificially sweetened . . . . 1 cup

Cheese: fat free . . . . 2 oz.

      low fat (3 gm fat or less per ounce) . . . . 1 1/2 oz.

STARCH EXCHANGES

(80 calories, 3 grams protein, 15 grams carbohydrate, 1 gram fat)

Starches are divided into two groups, grains and starchy vegetables, so you'll get all the benefits of the Food Guide Pyramid recommendation to eat 6–11 grain servings daily. Sample menu plans include at least six servings of grains, with extra starches chosen from either the grains or starchy vegetable group. When planning your own meals, choose at least six grains daily, then feel free to choose the rest of your starches from either grains or starches.

GRAINS (Choose at least six servings per day)

COUNT AS ONE GRAIN OR ONE STARCH:

Small bagel, English muffin, hot dog or
      hamburger roll . . . . 1/2 (1 oz.)

Bread: white, whole wheat, rye pumpernickel,
      multigrain, raisin . . . . 1 slice (1 oz.)

Pita (white or whole grain), corn tortilla,
      flour tortilla 1 (6-inch)

Small roll. . . . . 1 (1 oz.)

Cereal: Bran or cooked (oatmeal,
      Cream of Wheat) . . . . 1/2 cup

Cold flake cereal, unsweetened . . . . 3/4 cup

Frosted . . . . 1/2 cup

Grape Nuts, low-fat granola, muesli . . . . 1/4 cup

Cooked grains: Bulgur, grits, kasha,
        millet or pasta . . . . 1/2 cup

Rice, brown or white . . . . 1/3 cup

Dry cornmeal, flour, wheat germ . . . . 3 tablespoons

Graham crackers (2 1/2-inch square). 3

Matzos . . . . 3/4 oz.

Melba toast . . . . 4 slices

Oyster crackers 24

Snack chips (no-fat–added tortilla or potato) . . . . 3/4 oz.

Whole-wheat crackers (no fat added) . . . . 3/4 oz.

COUNT AS ONE GRAIN PLUS ONE FAT:

Biscuit, 2 1/2 inches. 1

Corn bread, 2-inch cube 1

Muffin, small 1

Pancake or waffle, 4 inches. 1

Taco shell. 2

STARCHY VEGETABLES

COUNT AS ONE STARCH:

Baked beans . . . . 1/3 cup

Corn, mixed vegetables, peas, plantain,
        mashed potato, sweet potato . . . . 1/2 cup

Corn on the cob . . . . 1 medium ear

Potato (baked or boiled)............................... I small

Acorn or butternut squash .... I cup

Beans (garbanzo, pinto, kidney, white, lima)
    or lentils.. 1/2 cup

Peas: split, black-eyed, yellow .... 1/2 cup

Miso... 3 tablespoons

VEGETABLES

(25 calories, 2 gm protein, 5 gm carbohydrate, 0 fat)

Only low-calorie vegetables are included in this list. Higher-calorie veggies are found in the starchy vegetables group. Each day, try to choose at least one dark green or deep orange fruit or vegetable to be sure to get your beta carotene. And choose at least one high in vitamin C, for healthy gums, quick wound healing and protection against heart disease and cancer. Vegetables marked (*) are high in vitamin C.

COUNT AS ONE VEGETABLE SERVING:

Alfalfa sprouts, artichoke, asparagus* .... 1/2 cup

Wax, green, Italian beans .... 1/2 cup

Bamboo shoots, bok choy*, snow peas,
    water chestnuts................................... 1/2 cup

Broccoli*, cauliflower*, Brussels sprouts* .... 1/2 cup

Carrots, celery, cucumber, radishes,
    mushrooms .... 1/2 cup

Greens*: collard, mustard, turnip, beet,
    kale, Swiss chard .... 1/2 cup

Green onion, leeks, onions .... 1/2 cup

Rutabaga or turnips .... 1/2 cup

Spinach, cooked .... 1/2 cup

Squash: patty pan, yellow, zucchini..................... 1/2 cup

Sweet pepper*: green, red, yellow . . . . 1/2 cup

Tomato* or vegetable juice . . . . 3/4 cup

Lettuce: endive, escarole, iceberg, green leaf,
     red leaf, romaine*, frisee, mesclun or
     spring mix, raw spinach* . . . . any amount

FRUIT

(60 calories, 0 protein, 15 gm carbohydrate, 0 fat)

Fruits and vegetables are loaded with fiber, and they're your best natural source of vitamin C and beta carotene. They're naturally low in calories, fat and sodium. But even too much fruit can add up to extra weight, so stick to your limits while you're trying to lose pounds and inches. Fruits marked (*) are high in vitamin C.

COUNT AS ONE FRUIT SERVING:

Apple, small. 1

Apple juice . . . . 1/2 cup

Apricots, fresh or dried. 2

Banana, small 1

Berries* . . . . 3/4 cup

Blended 100% fruit juice*. . . . . 1/3 cup

Cantaloupe*. . . . . 1 cup

Cherries 12

Figs, fresh or dried 2

Grapefruit* 1/2

Grapefruit juice* . . . . 1/2 cup

Grapes. 15

Grape juice. . . . . 1/3 cup

Honeydew melon*. . . . . 1 cup

Kiwifruit*. 1

Nectarine 1

Mandarin oranges* (juice pack) . . . . 3/4 cup

Mango* . . . . 1/2 cup

Orange* 1

Orange juice* . . . . 1/2 cup

Papaya* . . . . 1 cup

Peach 1

Pear, small 1

Pineapple, fresh or juice pack . . . . 1/2 cup

Pineapple juice . . . . 1/2 cup

Plums, small 2

Prunes 3

Prune juice . . . . 1/3 cup

Raisins . . . . 2 Tbsp

Strawberries*, whole . . . . 1 1/4 cups

Tangerines*, small 2

Watermelon* . . . . 1 1/4 cups

FATS

(50 calories, 0 protein, 0 carbohydrate, 5 gm fat)

Fats are divided into two groups, unsaturated and saturated. Calories are the same, but saturated fats clog your arteries and increase your risk of heart disease. But including some fat in your diet is necessary so you can absorb the fat-soluble vitamins from your food. Eating a little fat won't make you fat, as long as your total calories for the day are less than you spend. So use a little fat but stay within your limits, and choose mostly unsaturated fats for a healthy heart!

COUNT AS ONE FAT SERVING: UNSATURATED

Avocado (average size) 1/8

Oil: canola, olive, peanut, corn, safflower,

soybean, sesame, walnut. . . . . 1 tsp

Olives: black . . . . 8 large

stuffed green . . . . 10 large

Nuts: almonds, cashews, peanuts, pecans. . . . . 1/4 oz.

Peanut butter . . . . 2 tsp

Sesame seeds, pumpkin seeds. . . . . 1 Tbsp

Margarine . . . . 1 tsp

low fat. . . . . 1 Tbsp

Mayonnaise . . . . 1 tsp

low fat. . . . . 1 Tbsp

COUNT AS ONE FAT SERVING: SATURATED

Cooked bacon. . . . . 1 slice

Butter . . . . 1 tsp

reduced fat. . . . . 1 Tbsp

Half-and-half . . . . 2 Tbsp

Cream cheese . . . . 1 Tbsp

reduced fat. . . . . 2 Tbsp

Sour cream . . . . 2 Tbsp

reduced fat. . . . . 3 Tbsp

CRAVE STOPPERS
THAT HIT THE SPOT

How many afternoons have you watched the clock strike three (the snacking hour) and said, "I need something chocolate!" It is completely natural for your body to crave specific foods. Denying yourself isn't necessary, and can later lead to binges that put on unwanted pounds. But remember, it only takes a little to satisfy the craving.

So be prepared. These planned afternoon treats average about 100 calories, and their fat and sugar have been calculated into your healthy eating plan.

Take control of temptation with portion-right treats that hit the spot!

IF YOU WANT CHOCOLATE, TRY . . .

1/2 cup 1% chocolate milk
1 packet low-fat hot-chocolate mix
2 fat-free chocolate cookies
18 chocolate Teddy grahams
2 chocolate rice cakes
1 1/2 tablespoons chocolate chips
1 chocolate sorbet bar
3/4 cup Dannon Light chocolate frozen yogurt

IF YOU WANT SOMETHING CREAMY, TRY . . .

1/2 cup fat-free ice cream
1/2 cup skim-milk pudding
3/4 cup applesauce
iced cappuccino made with skim milk
1 small banana
1 small red-skinned potato
1/2 cup spicy black bean dip
1/2 cup cereal with 1/2 cup skim milk

IF YOU WANT SOMETHING SWEET, TRY . . .

2 fruit Newtons, any flavor
frozen fruit-juice bar
3 fortune cookies
3 ginger snaps
small piece of angel food cake
10 Lifesavers
8 animal crackers

IF YOU WANT SOMETHING SALTY
AND CRUNCHY TRY . . .

1 oz. pretzels
1 1/2 oz. fat-free potato chips
1 oz. no-fat-added tortilla chips
9 saltine crackers
4 cups lowfat microwave popcorn
5 no-fat-added whole wheat crackers

To get you started, I've created a week's worth of menus using a wide variety of choices from all the pyramid food groups. You'll find the menu on the left, with serving sizes that are right for each of our three calorie-level diets. All the work has been done for you. You'll find exciting, delicious meals to speed you on your way to a trimmer, healthier body.

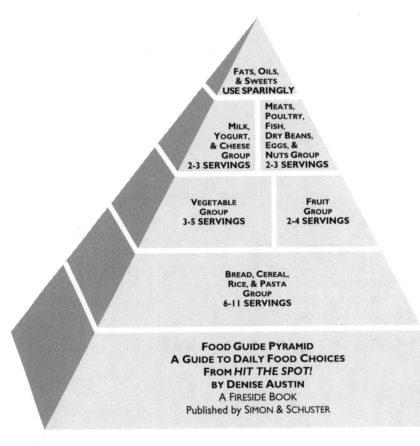

FATS, OILS,
& SWEETS
USE SPARINGLY

MILK,
YOGURT,
& CHEESE
GROUP
2-3 SERVINGS

MEATS,
POULTRY,
FISH,
DRY BEANS,
EGGS, &
NUTS GROUP
2-3 SERVINGS

VEGETABLE
GROUP
3-5 SERVINGS

FRUIT
GROUP
2-4 SERVINGS

BREAD, CEREAL,
RICE, & PASTA
GROUP
6-11 SERVINGS

**FOOD GUIDE PYRAMID
A GUIDE TO DAILY FOOD CHOICES
FROM *HIT THE SPOT!*
BY DENISE AUSTIN**
A FIRESIDE BOOK
Published by SIMON & SCHUSTER

Sample Meals • Day 1

	1350	1600	2200
BREAKFAST			
skim milk	I cup	I cup	I cup
flake cereal	2 1/4 cups	2 1/4 cups	2 1/4 cups
whole-wheat toast		I slice	2 slices
margarine		2 teaspoons	2 teaspoons
grapefruit juice	1/2 cup	1/2 cup	1/2 cup
LUNCH			
SANDWICH:			
rye bread	2 slices	2 slices	2 slices
lean ham	2 ounces	2 ounces	2 ounces
lowfat cheese	2 slices	2 slices	2 slices
lettuce and tomato	I serving	I serving	I serving
mayonnaise	2 teaspoons	2 teaspoons	2 teaspoons
raw carrot nuggets		1/2 cup	1/2 cup
low-fat tortilla chips			I 1/2 ounces
fresh peach	I	I	I
SNACK			
CRAVE STOPPER:			
chocolate skim-milk pudding	1/2 cup	1/2 cup	1/2 cup
ripe banana	none	one small	one small
DINNER			
ORIENTAL STIR FRY:			
turkey breast cutlet	2 ounces	2 ounces	2 ounces
mixed veggies	I cup	I cup	I 1/2 cups
sesame oil	2 teaspoons	2 teaspoons	4 teaspoons
mandarin oranges			1/2 cup
Brown or white rice	2/3 cup	2/3 cup	I cup

Spray a heavy nonstick skillet with cooking spray. Over medium heat, sauté cubed turkey breast until cooked through. Stir in one teaspoon chopped garlic and 1/2 teaspoon chopped fresh ginger. Quickly add vegetables. Include snow peas, water chestnuts, mung bean sprouts, bamboo shoots and chopped green onions. Cook vegetables, stirring constantly, until tender crisp. If necessary, add a small amount of defatted chicken broth to prevent sticking. Toss vegetables with allowed sesame oil and mandarin oranges. Add soy sauce to taste. Serve over rice.

Sample Meals • Day 2

	1350	1600	2200
BREAKFAST			
Sandwich:			
lowfat cheese	1.5 oz.	1.5 oz.	1.5 oz.
English muffin	1 sandwich size	2 regular size	2 sandwich size
fresh pear	one small	one small	one small
LUNCH			
SANDWICH:			
Lettuce and tomato	1 serving	1 serving	1 serving
multigrain bread	2 slices	2 slices	2 slices
lean roast beef	2 oz.	2 oz.	2 oz.
mayonnaise	1 tsp	1 tsp	1 tsp
pretzels	none	none	1.5 oz.
nonfat yogurt	1 cup	1 cup	1 cup
kiwifruit	one	one	one
SNACK			
CRAVE STOPPER	3 ginger snaps	3 ginger snaps	3 ginger snaps
Pineapple juice	none	1/2 cup	1/2 cup
DINNER			
grilled tuna steaks	2 oz.	2 oz.	2 oz.
sweet rainbow salsa	1/2 cup	1/2 cup	1/2 cup

herbed			
sandwich roll	one	one	one
mesclun salad	2 cups	2 cups	2 cups
olive oil	I tsp	I tsp	2 tsp
grated carrots			
and mushrooms	none	none	I cup
pinenuts	none	none	I Tbsp
baked beans	none	none	1/3 cup
fresh mango	none	none	1/2 cup

Brush tuna steaks with I tablespoon hickory-flavored barbecue sauce. Grill over hot coals until steaks flake easily when tested with a fork, about 2 minutes per side. Place tuna steak on a sandwich roll. Top with sweet rainbow salsa.

Sweet rainbow salsa: In a heavy nonstick skillet over medium heat, cook one medium onion, cut in eighths and thickly sliced. Stir constantly until onion is tender, adding a little water to prevent burning. Add 3 tablespoons balsamic vinegar, 2 medium tomatoes (peeled, seeded, and chopped) and one each sweet green and sweet yellow peppers (seeded and chopped). Cook, stirring, about 5 minutes. Stir in 2 tablespoons chopped fresh cilantro, I tablespoon chopped fresh basil and one small, overripe banana, chopped. Serve warm or chilled.

Toss mesclun salad with allowed olive oil, carrots, mushrooms and pine nuts.

Sample Meals • Day 3

	1350	1600	2200
BREAKFAST			
nonfat yogurt	8 oz.	8 oz.	8 oz.
lowfat granola	3/4 cup	I cup	I 1/4 cup
fresh blueberries	3/4 cup	3/4 cup	3/4 cup
chopped walnuts	none	8 halves	8 halves
LUNCH			
Sandwich:			
small whole			
wheat pita	one	one	two
sliced turkey breast	2 oz.	2 oz.	2 oz.

lowfat cheese	1.5 oz.	1.5 oz.	1.5 oz.
alfalfa sprouts	1/2 cup	1/2 cup	1/2 cup
romaine	large leaf	large leaf	large leaf
tomato, sliced	none	one small	one small
olive oil	2 tsp	2 tsp	2 tsp
plums, small	2	2	2

SNACK

CRAVE STOPPER:

fat-free potato chips	1 1/2 oz.	1 1/2 oz.	1 1/2 oz.
Grapefruit juice	none	1/2 cup	1/2 cup

DINNER

TORTILLA SCRAMBLE:

chopped veggies	1 cup	1 cup	1 cup
egg whites	4	4	4
6-inch tortilla	1	1	2
black beans	1/2 cup	1/2 cup	1/2 cup
reduced-fat sour cream	3 Tbsp	3 Tbsp	3 Tbsp
fresh pineapple	none	none	1/2 cup
leafy salad	large	large	large
corn oil	1 tsp	1 tsp	1 tsp

Coat a heavy nonstick skillet with a burst of cooking spray. Stir in chopped vegetables, including 1/4 cup each sweet red and green peppers, 1/2 cup diced onions, 1 small jalapeno pepper (diced) and 1/4 teaspoon each chopped garlic and ground cumin. Cook over medium heat, stirring occasionally, until vegetables begin to wilt. While vegetables are cooking, combine egg whites with 1/4 cup water, then beat with a wire whisk until whites begin to foam slightly. Pour over vegetables. Cover pan and reduce heat to low. Allow egg mixture to stand, without stirring, until cooked through, about 5 minutes. Remove omelet to plate.

Place tortilla on plate, top with warm beans and sour cream, then roll.

Serve with leafy salad blended with chopped fresh cilantro, and a dressing made with corn oil, red wine vinegar, salt and pepper to taste.

	1350	1600	2200
BREAKFAST			
graham crackers	3 (2 1/2-in.sq)	6 squares	6 squares
peanut butter	none	2 tsp	2 tsp
Frosted Miniwheats	I cup	I cup	I 1/2 cups
skim milk	I cup	I cup	I cup
grapefruit	1/2	1/2	1/2
LUNCH			
CALIFORNIA GRILLED CHICKEN SALAD:			
tossed salad	large	large	large
olive oil	I tsp	I tsp	I tsp
grilled chicken	2 oz.	2 oz.	2 oz.
lowfat Jarlsberg	I 1/2 oz.	I 1/2 oz.	I1/2 oz.
avocado	1/8	1/8	1/8
whole-wheat crackers	I 1/2 oz.	I 1/2 oz.	3 oz.
nectarine	I	I	I
SNACK			
CRAVE STOPPER:			
fat-free ice cream	1/2 cup	1/2 cup	1/2 cup
cantaloupe	none	I cup	I cup
DINNER			
PASTA ITALIANO:			
olive oil	2 tsp	2 tsp	4 tsp
tomato sauce	1/2 cup	1/2 cup	3/4 cup
cannellini beans	1/2 cup	1/2 cup	1/2 cup
steamed broccoli	1/2 cup	1/2 cup	3/4 cup
leafy salad	2 cups	2 cups	2 cups
apricots	none	none	two

In a heavy, nonstick saucepan, sauté one teaspoon chopped garlic in allowed olive oil until garlic is soft but not browned. Stir in tomato sauce. Add 1/8 teaspoon aniseseed, a dash of cayenne pepper, and two fresh basil leaves, thinly sliced (or 1/2 teaspoon dried basil). Simmer two to three minutes. Stir in beans. Cover pan and simmer two to three more minutes, or until beans are heated through. Serve over fettucine noodles.

Steam broccoli with 1/4 teaspoon dried oregano. Season with salt, pepper and a squeeze of fresh lemon. Toss one cup each romaine and spinach leaves with fat-free Italian dressing.

Sample Meals • Day 5

	1350	1600	2200
BREAKFAST			
bagel	3 oz.	4 oz.	5 oz.
lowfat Muenster			
cheese	1 1/2 oz.	1 1/2 oz.	1 1/2 oz.
orange juice	1/2 cup	1/2 cup	1/2 cup
fat	none	none	none
LUNCH			
EGG SALAD:			
hard-boiled egg	1	1	1
mayonnaise	2 tsp	2 tsp	2 tsp
celery	1/4 cup	1/4 cup	1/4 cup
sliced radishes	1/4 cup	1/4 cup	1/4 cup
chopped cucumber	1/4 cup	1/4 cup	1/4 cup
whole-wheat pita	one 6-inch	one 6-inch	one large
romaine	large leaf	large leaf	large leaf
vanilla nonfat			
yogurt	8 oz.	8 oz.	8 oz.
fresh raspberries	3/4 cup	3/4 cup	3/4 cup
SNACK			
CRAVE STOPPER:			
lowfat microwave			
popcorn	4 cups	4 cups	4 cups
grape juice	none	1/3 cup	1/3 cup

DINNER

WINE-POACHED SALMON:

salmon	2 oz.	2 oz.	2 oz.
red-skinned potato	I small	I small	2 small
margarine	I tsp	2 tsp	4 tsp
small dinner roll	I	I	I
Greek green beans	I cup	I cup	I 1/2 cups
onion	1/4 cup	1/4 cup	1/4 cup
fresh blueberries	none	none	3/4 cup

In a heavy, nonstick skillet, place salmon, skin side down. Pour enough red wine over the salmon to almost cover. Simmer over medium heat until salmon is cooked through and flakes easily when tested with a fork, and wine is almost gone. Season with salt and pepper to taste.

Microwave red-skinned potato on high until cooked through, about 5 to 8 minutes. Season with margarine and fresh chives.

Greek green beans: In a heavy skillet coated with cooking spray, cook 1/4 cup chopped onion until soft. Stir in 1/2 teaspoon chopped garlic, one small tomato (peeled, seeded and chopped) and 1/2 teaspoon oregano. Cook, stirring often, for 3 minutes. Wash 1/2 pound green beans, then break into 2-inch pieces. Stir into tomato mixture. Cook, covered, until tender, about 5 minutes.

Sample Meals • Day 6

	1350	1600	2200
BREAKFAST			
oatmeal (cooked)	I cup	I cup	I 1/2 cups
raisins	2 Tbsp	2 Tbsp	2 Tbsp
chopped pecans	none	1/2 oz.	1/2 oz.
whole-wheat toast	I slice	2 slices	2 slices
1% milk	8 oz.	8 oz.	8 oz.
LUNCH			
very lowfat hot dog	I	I	I
fat-free cheese	2 oz.	2 oz.	2 oz.
hot dog roll	I	I	I

shredded cabbage and carrots	1/2 cup	1/2 cup	1 cup
fat-free coleslaw dressing	1 Tbsp	1 Tbsp	1 Tbsp
watermelon	1 1/4 cups	1 1/4 cups	1 1/4 cups
fat-free potato chips	none	none	1 1/2 oz.

SNACK

CRAVE STOPPER:

Chocolate Teddy grahams	18	18	18
Blended fruit juice	none	1/3 cup	1/3 cup

DINNER

DIJON CHICKEN:

chicken	2 oz.	2 oz.	2 oz.
mashed potatoes	1/2 cup	1/2 cup	1 cup
reduced-fat sour cream	3 Tbsp	3 Tbsp	3 Tbsp
dinner roll	1	1	1
margarine	1 tsp	1 tsp	1 tsp
cooked spinach	1 cup	1 cup	1 cup
yellow raisins	none	none	2 Tbsp
olive oil	none	none	2 tsp
red-leaf lettuce	2 cups	2 cups	2 cups
fat-free Catalina dressing	1 Tbsp	1 Tbsp	1 Tbsp
artichoke hearts	none	none	two

Brush both sides of a small, boneless, skinless chicken breast with Dijon mustard. Place on broiler pan covered with aluminum foil lightly coated with cooking spray. Broil 4 minutes per side, or until chicken is cooked through and juices run clear (not pink) when chicken is pierced with a fork.

Whip hot mashed potatoes with sour cream, salt and pepper to taste and enough skim milk to create the thickness you prefer.

Thoroughly wash fresh spinach. Shake off excess water, and place spinach in a heavy pot with a tight-fitting lid. The water clinging to the spinach should be just enough for successful cooking. Dust spinach with a pinch of ground nutmeg and a pinch of salt. If allowed, add raisins. Cook over medium heat until spinach is just wilted. If allowed, toss with olive oil. (One pound of fresh spinach makes about two cups of cooked spinach.)

Toss red leaf lettuce with salad dressing. Garnish with artichoke hearts, if allowed.

Sample Meals • Day 7

	1350	1600	2200
BREAKFAST			
waffles (lowfat)	2	4	5
vanilla nonfat			
yogurt	8 oz.	8 oz.	8 oz.
cinnamon			
applesauce	1/2 cup	1/2 cup	1/2 cup
LUNCH			
SANDWICH:			
water-packed			
tuna	2 oz.	2 oz.	2 oz.
mayonnaise	2 tsp	2 tsp	2 tsp
chopped celery	1 tablespoon	1 tablespoon	1 tablespoon
lettuce leaf			
pumpernickel			
bread	2 slices	2 slices	2 slices
vegetable soup	1/2 cup vegetables	1 cup vegetables	2 cups vegetables
pretzels	none	none	1 1/2 oz.
fat-free yogurt	8 oz.	8 oz.	8 oz.
fresh cherries	12	12	12
SNACK			
CRAVE STOPPER:			
Dannon Light			
frozen yogurt	3/4 cup	3/4 cup	3/4 cup
fresh			
strawberries	none	1 1/4 cups	1 1/4 cups

	1350	1600	2200
DINNER			
ON THE GRILL:			
pork tenderloin	**2 oz.**	**2 oz.**	**2 oz.**
confetti veggies	**I cup**	**I cup**	**I cup**
olive oil	**I/2 tsp**	**I/2 tsp**	**I/2 tsp**
corn on the cob	**I medium**	**I medium**	**I medium**
dinner roll	**one small**	**one small**	**two small**
butter or			
margarine	**I/2 tsp**	**I/2 tsp**	**2 I/2 tsp**
watermelon	**none**	**none**	**I I/4 cups**

Brush a whole pork tenderloin with one tablespoon barbecue sauce (any flavor). Grill over coals or under broiler, turning every 5 minutes until done, usually about 20 minutes. Be careful not to overcook, as pork will become very dry. Slice tenderloin into two-ounce portions.

Combine halved baby eggplant, 2-inch chunks of green and yellow squash, baby carrots and pearl onions in quantities large enough to create one-cup servings for each guest. For each serving, add 1 teaspoon chopped garlic, 1/2 teaspoon dried rosemary, and 1/2 teaspoon olive oil. Mix thoroughly, then spread in a single layer in grill basket or on broiler pan. Cook about 5 minutes, or until vegetables begin to soften and char slightly. Toss cooked vegetables with 1 tablespoon balsamic vinegar per serving. Serve hot or chilled.

ACCELERATE THE FAT-BURNING PROCESS . . . IT INCREASES YOUR METABOLISM.

FOOD ISN'T THE ENEMY. SITTING STILL IS!

ADDITIONAL RECIPES

Here are ten great recipes to give variety to your daily meal plan, because if you are like me, you're always looking for quick, low-fat, easy dishes! All of these recipes are simple. You don't have to be a gourmet chef. They are low in fat, and taste great! You can have an entire meal on the table in less than 20 minutes!

Bon Appétit! . . . food is fabulous!

EASY CHICKEN SOUP

1/4 cup pearl barley

1 cup chopped onion

4 cups reduced-sodium chicken broth

1 cup dry white wine

1 cup fat-free tomato sauce

1 tablespoon dried tarragon

1/2 teaspoon salt

1/2 teaspoon pepper

2 raw carrots, sliced

1 cup sliced zucchini

1 cup sliced yellow squash

1 8-ounce can yellow corn

2 large chicken breasts, cut into one-inch strips

Cook pearl barley according to package directions and keep warm. Place chopped onion in heavy, nonstick saucepan, and cook over low heat until clear and tender (about 3 minutes). Stir in chicken broth, white wine, tomato sauce, tarragon and salt and pepper. Cover and bring to a boil. Stir in carrots and cook 7 minutes. Add zucchini and yellow squash, yellow corn, well-drained, and chicken breasts. Cook 5 minutes. For each serving, place one fourth of the cooked barley in a large soup bowl. Top with one-fourth of the soup (about 1 1/2 cups).

COLD PEANUT NOODLES WITH MIXED VEGETABLES

3/4 cup cooked fat-free ramen noodles

1 cup raw spinach

1/2 cup chopped cucumber

1 small grated carrot

1 chopped green onion

1/4 cup canned chick peas

2 teaspoons peanut butter

1 tablespoon teriyaki sauce

1/2 teaspoon minced garlic

Toss noodles with spinach, cucumber, carrot, green onion and chick peas. Add a dressing made of peanut butter thinned with 2 tablespoons water and teriyaki sauce and minced garlic. Toss until noodles and vegetables are coated with sauce. Serve immediately or chill.

SHRIMP WITH AVOCADO

1 medium red-skinned potato

1/8 soft, ripe avocado

1 teaspoon fresh lemon juice

2 ounces chopped, cooked, peeled, deveined shrimp

2 fresh sliced mushrooms

1 tablespoon fresh or 1 teaspoon dried chopped chives

Seafood seasoning (such as Old Bay) to taste

Bake or microwave potato until done. Meanwhile, mash avocado with lemon juice. Combine with deveined shrimp, mushrooms, chives and seafood seasoning, such as Old Bay, to taste. Stuff filling into split, cooked potato.

HONEY-SESAME PORK

3-ounce slice pork tenderloin

2 teaspoons honey

1 teaspoon reduced-sodium soy sauce

3/4 teaspoon sesame seeds

1 cup cooked white rice

1 cup frozen Chinese vegetables, cooked

Brown a pork tenderloin in a nonstick skillet lightly coated with cooking spray. Roll cooked pork in honey mixed with soy sauce, then roll in sesame seeds. Lay on foil coated with cooking spray and broil until lightly browned. Serve over rice mixed with vegetables.

CHEESE VEGETABLE PIZZA

1 individual Boboli pizza shell

1/2 cup fat-free tomato sauce

dash ground cayenne pepper

1/8 teaspoon anise seed

2 whole canned artichoke hearts, cut in half

2 fresh mushrooms, sliced

1 ounce reduced-fat mozzarella cheese

Top pizza shell with tomato sauce seasoned with cayenne pepper and anise seed. Add artichoke hearts, mushrooms, and mozzarella cheese. Bake for eight to ten minutes at 450 degrees.

EAT BREAKFAST LIKE A KING,
LUNCH LIKE A QUEEN, AND
DINNER LIKE A PAUPER.
PUT A CURFEW ON YOUR KITCHEN . . .
DON'T EAT ANYTHING FOR THREE HOURS
BEFORE BEDTIME.

SAVORY CHICKEN SAUTÉ

Lemony Rice (see below)

4 boneless, skinless chicken breast
    halves (about 1 pound)

3 tablespoons olive oil

1 large onion, sliced

2 cloves garlic, minced

1 tablespoon chopped fresh rosemary
    or 1 1/2 teaspoons dried rose-
    mary, crushed

1/2 cup chicken broth

4 medium red Florida grapefruit,
    peeled and segmented

Salt and pepper

Prepare Lemony Rice. Meanwhile, in large skillet over medium heat, sauté chicken in hot oil 4 minutes; turn chicken over and add onion. Cover and cook 3 minutes longer, stirring occasionally. Add garlic, rosemary, and broth. Cover and cook until onion is crisp-tender, about 5 minutes longer, stirring occasionally. Stir in grapefruit; season with salt and pepper to taste. Serve with hot Lemony Rice.

LEMONY RICE

1 3/4 cups chicken broth

1/4 cup fresh lemon juice

1 cup rice

1 tablespoon chopped fresh parsley

In medium saucepan, combine broth, lemon juice. Bring to boil; stir in rice. Reduce heat to low, cover and simmer 20 minutes or until all liquid is absorbed and rice is tender. Stir in parsley.

Yields: 4 servings.

COMPOSED FRUIT SALAD

Lemon Poppy Seed Dressing
(see below)

Butter lettuce leaves

1/2 small honeydew melon, peeled
and sliced lengthwise

3 medium white and/or red Florida
grapefruit, peeled and sliced
crosswise (about 1/4-inch thick),
then each slice halved

2 oranges, peeled and segmented

1 ripe papaya, peeled, seeded
and sliced

LEMON POPPY SEED DRESSING

In small bowl, combine 2/3 cup plain low-fat yogurt, 1 tablespoon fresh lemon juice, 1 tablespoon honey and 1/4 teaspoon poppy seeds. Yields: 4–5 servings. Prepare Lemon Poppy Seed Dressing; cover and refrigerate if making ahead.

To serve, on 4 individual plates, arrange butter lettuce leaves. Divide fruit evenly among plates, arranging the pieces attractively. Drizzle dressing on each salad.

FRUIT, NUT AND CHEESE SALAD

Balsamic Vinaigrette (see below)

6 cups torn mixed greens (spinach,
butter lettuce, curly endive)

3 medium red Florida grapefruit,
peeled and segmented

1 cup red grapes, halved

1/2 small red onion, thinly sliced

1/4 cup coarsely chopped walnuts,
toasted

4 ounces blue cheese, crumbled

Prepare Balsamic Vinaigrette. In large salad bowl, combine remaining ingredients. Pour vinaigrette over salad and toss well.

BALSAMIC VINAIGRETTE

In small bowl, whisk together 1/4 cup balsamic vinegar*, 2 tablespoons olive oil (or vegetable oil), 2 tablespoons honey and 1 tablespoon Dijon mustard.

Yields: 6 servings.

*1/4 cup freshly squeezed grapefruit juice may be substituted.

HIT THE SPOT BLENDER DRINKS

Here are two of my favorite blender drinks. These recipes are great for breakfast, especially if you are in a hurry, as a healthy snack or an afternoon exercise cooler. They are refreshing and fat free!

ICY FRUIT NECTAR

This recipe is easy and quick to make. If you use frozen fruit, it makes preparation even quicker and easier, and cleanup is a snap!

Makes 3 cups

3/4 cup very cold apple juice

2 cups frozen (no sugar added) or fresh fruit such as peaches, strawberries or other combination

2 packets Equal or more to taste

2 teaspoons lemon juice

3 ice cubes

Place ingredients in blender and process on low until ice begins to blend into mixture. Increase speed to high and process until smooth. Pour into chilled glasses and enjoy!

Nutrition information per 1 cup serving: Calories 90, Fat 0

STRAWBERRY FREEZE

This recipe provides a great calcium boost to your daily diet. Your kids will love it, too . . . mine do!

Makes 3 cups

1/2 cup plain nonfat yogurt

2 tablespoons nonfat dry milk powder

1/2 cup orange juice

1 1/4 cups frozen (no sugar added) or fresh strawberries

1/2 medium banana, ripe, cut into chunks

2 packets Equal or more to taste

dash of vanilla extract

3 ice cubes

Place ingredients in blender and process on low until ice begins to blend into mixture. Increase speed to high and process until smooth. Pour into chilled glasses and enjoy!

Nutrition information per 1 cup serving: Calories 90, Fat 0

HIDE THE SPOT

SUPER SOLUTIONS TO SLIMLINE YOUR FIGURE

How many times have you gone to your closet in search of something to wear, only to choose one of two outfits: the new black one or the old black one?

Women of all shapes and sizes need help in camouflaging certain trouble spots, but a wardrobe consisting entirely of black is not the answer.

As we have seen through much of the history of fashion, even beautiful women went to painful extremes to accentuate the positive and hide the negative. Think of Scarlett O'Hara cinching her waist, and Victorian women with their bustiers and bustles.

Fortunately for us, there are painless ways to disguise a thick waistline, wide hips and flabby arms, and hide those areas which make us cringe when we look in the mirror. Dressing your best is an instant boost to your confidence, and I want you to learn to perk up your appearance everyday.

My worst spots are my thighs: They are short and muscular. Great for gymnastics, but sometimes difficult when it comes to choosing clothes. I look for softly pleated pants or skirts that create an illusion of a slimmer silhouette. Anything that tightly hugs the body will accentuate the problem area. I stay away from Spandex pants unless I'm working out.

I have a small bustline, so I often wear a padded bra to give extra lift. Wide belts accentuate my waist and I adore low-cut tailored jackets. Whenever I appear on television, I try to wear a lighter top and a darker bottom. I want to look larger on top and smaller around my thighs. Remember: Lighter-colored clothing will always draw the eye.

My sisters and friends always ask me for advice on choosing clothes that will help them appear slimmer. Here are some stylish solutions that will instantly streamline your figure, as well as styles that should be avoided.

One exercise: Take your own before and after Polaroid pictures with a friend. Try wearing something from the avoid category, and then switching to the what-to-look-for choices. Compare the snapshots, front and back. You'll see the difference instantly!

DO YOU HAVE A THICK WAISTLINE OR POUCHY TUMMY?

Mid-section miracles don't necessarily happen through costly surgery. Instant results can be achieved simply by choosing the right styles.

You don't have to wear a designer size 6 to find flattering, fashionable clothes. There are many styles that can complement a fuller figure. Colorful boxy jackets or double-breasted styles that fall just below your hips are a good choice when paired with soft skirts or tapered pants. You should stay away from clingy knits. Sweaters that fall below the tummy and hips are a good choice. You don't have to avoid bright colors: Dark sapphire blue, emerald green or ruby red are a good alternative to basic black.

Fabric weight is crucial: choose lighter, thinner materials that drape elegantly, such as silk and rayon.

You can also instantly deflate a prominent tummy by choosing a vertically striped vest or blouse, which acts as an optical illusion: A tapered top can trim inches off your middle.

Just because you've gained a few pounds doesn't mean you can't wear a belt. Just make sure it's the same color as your dress or outfit since it then won't disrupt the vertical line.

If you want to instantly whittle your middle, try following these suggestions.

What to avoid:

- **Gathered skirts: The fabric will bulge just where you don't want it to: at or below the waist.**

- **Jackets belted at the waist: too bulky.**

- **Skimpy, tight tops.**

- **Horizontal stripes and designs.**

- **Fly-front closings.**

What to look for:

- **Dresses with Empire bodices: They draw attention up and away from the waist.**

- **Any V neckline: The deeper the V, the longer the line.**

- **Tailored pants with a classic fit. Narrow legs and side or back zippers are also a good choice. Baggy pants never fool anyone.**

- **Narrow belts . . . forget the wide ones.**

- **A polo sweater with a banded bottom covers tummy bulges and draws attention upward.**

- **Shirtdresses camouflage a thick middle.**

- **A-line skirts will create the illusion of a nipped-in middle.**

- **Sheath dress with matching jacket: A single color is most slimming. The dress covers a thick waist, and the jacket hides hips and rear end.**

- **Control-top pantyhose: a must!**

DO YOU HAVE BIG THIGHS?

I've been called by that dreaded nickname: Thunder Thighs. It hurt my feelings as much as it hurts yours. This is my problem area, and it is a result of years of gymnastics, not to mention my genetic predisposition. I've learned a few tricks to streamline my thighs, even in short skirts.

To make my legs look longer and leaner, I wear at least a two-inch heel; they do wonders for my legs. If you have thick thighs, it's important to have toned calf muscles—this will balance the shape of your leg. Heels accentuate the shape of your calf.

When choosing a bathing suit, I look for a high-cut leg that creates the illusion of a longer, leaner thigh. It's lengthening, and slimming. Plus, it's sexier. I tend to wear darker colors on the legs, and I love the new midriff styles, which draw attention to my best feature: a tight tummy.

The secret is to accent the positive! The best way I have found to trim my thighs is to wear a slim skirt that barely skims the lower body. I have to buy a size larger than usual to get a proper fit, but I promise you'll love the slimmer silhouette.

I have trouble buying blue jeans because the legs tend to be skin tight. I always buy jeans with flat, classic-front pockets. Side pockets accentuate hips. I never try to squeeze into jeans that are too small. Nothing is less appealing than a woman who looks like a sausage encased in denim.

What to avoid:

- Carrying your pocketbook at the hip level; adjust the strap so it doesn't hit the widest part of your hips. Also, try carrying a clutch under your arm. It will draw attention away from your middle and to the bustline.

- Bright-colored bottoms; the eye focuses there first.

- Clingy fabrics and bulky knits.

- Dropped-waist dresses: They make anyone look frumpy, and draw attention to the thighs.

- Hip-huggers.

- Contrasting colored belts: They create a distinct horizontal line, dividing you into two blocks.

- Skip neckties, long necklaces, and tight tops that emphasize the fact that your hips are wider than your shoulders.

- Ankle-strap shoes: they shorten your leg. To flatter your leg, your heels should taper or curve. Avoid chunky heels.

- Tight shorts.

What to look for:

- Brightly colored tops: They distract from your not-so-perfect hips and thighs.

- Boat-neck tops: They make your shoulders look wider and balance the width of your lower body.

- Long, drop earrings: They draw attention to your face and can create vertical lines.

- Simply shaped shoes with a bit of a heel, preferably tapered.

- Soft skirts which graze the body, not hug it. Think slim, not tight.

- Loose pants with full-cut legs; instant slimmer.

- Waist-length tops, even ones with diagonal stripes which lead the eye up and away from your hips.

- Wrap panel sweaters, which create a V neck.

- Below the hip, narrow jackets. Avoid double-breasted or wide lapel styles. They create "fattening" horizontal lines.

- Softly padded shoulders; they balance a hip-heavy torso, giving the illusion of a near-perfect figure.

DO YOU HAVE GLUTEUS TOO MAXIMUS?

The most common complaint among my friends is the fact that they are unhappy with the size of their tushes. No matter how much we exercise, we still need a bit of camouflaging in that area. Especially as we grow older and the force of gravity kicks in.

So, let's kick butt!

A toned, tight bottom is the ultimate goal. But for our less-than-perfect rears, there are many ways to hide your flaws and flatter your derriere. It's not just the size; a flat, untoned bottom can be just as unattractive as an oversized one.

Skirts may not be a problem as much as pants. To get the fit you want, make sure the waistband, fly, pleats, and pockets lie flat. There shouldn't be any pulling across your fanny, tummy or crotch.

What to avoid:

- Tucking in your blouse: it not only bunches up more fabric where you don't want it, cinching in the waist accentuates your rear view.

- Cropped tops and jackets.

- Jeans or pants with back detailing.

- Covering a skirt with a sweater; it only adds more inches.

- **Bulky fabrics.**

- **A skimpy top with pants; your bottom half will always look wider.**

- **Brights on the bottom.**

- **Leggings or cigarette pants.**

What to look for:

- **Softly fitted jackets that cover your rear end.**

- **Full cut, wide-leg pants.**

- **Straight-leg pants paired with long tunics.**

- **Sheath dresses.**

- **Longer blazers.**

- **Bias-cut dresses do wonders in covering a pear-shaped figure. Vertical seams elongate the line of the body.**

- **Colorful scarves. An optical trick; eyes are drawn immediately to interesting patterns.**

- **Dark pantyhose and shoes; any figure looks longer and leaner with a continuous vertical line.**

- **Try this no-fail, super slimming outfit: A long nonclingy sweater with a slim skirt or pants. A-line skirts can also conceal a large rear end. Pants should hang straight from the hip to the ankle.**

DO YOU HAVE LARGE, WIDE HIPS?

My sister, who is so beautiful, has been cursed with less-than-perfect hips. Diet and exercise have helped, but she has also learned several tricks to slim her hips by choosing the right clothes.

She avoids tight, form-fitting styles which only call attention to her pear shape. She looks best in straight dresses and jackets in the same color or tone. Her silhouette looks long and lean from any angle. You too can learn how to look slimmer instantly with these simple solutions.

What to avoid:

- **Any top which hits you at the hip level. Stay away from drop waist dresses.**

- **Bright-colored leggings, unless covered with a matching, lean top that doesn't cling.**

- **Anything sloppy that clings to your hips.**

- **Pleated skirts.**

- **Anything that zips up the side.**

What to look for:

- **Skirts that are lined: they are less likely to cling.**

- **One-piece bodysuits that form a lean line, topped with a longer vest or tailored jacket.**

- **Color: Go for dark shades below the waistline, keep lighter shades and patterns on top.**

- **Body-shaping pantyhose with extra Lycra.**

- **Shirts in fabrics that drape easily.**

- **To draw attention upward, wear a large piece of jewelry at the neck or shoulder.**

DO YOU HAVE FLABBY ARMS? SAGGING BREASTS?

I know most of us care about hiding the lower half of our body, but it's important to think about the shape of your arms.

You know you have flabby upper arms if, when you wave goodbye, the skin under your biceps keeps jiggling.

What to avoid:

- **Tank tops and capped sleeves: Choose loose fitting sleeves which stop approximately three inches above the elbow.**

- **Anything skintight around your upper arm will only exaggerate the abundance of loose flesh.**

What to look for:

- **If you're feeling sexy, off the shoulder tops with longer sleeves accentuate your neck and bustline and draw attention away from your arms.**

- **Dropped-shoulder tops are best: Choose silky, flowing fabrics for a soft draped effect.**

Sagging breasts can be controlled with a great underwire bra. There are so many choices, and the newer styles are even more comfortable than before.

If you are busty, choose a bra with diagonal seaming, which helps equalize breasts and gives super support. Also, avoid wide belts that shorten your upper body and call attention to your chest.

Low-cut dresses with a modest amount of cleavage are sexier than skintight turtlenecks with no definition.

DO YOU HAVE A FLAT CHEST?

Nobody ever accused me of being stacked.

I was not blessed with a well-endowed chest. It has never made me feel inadequate in any way, but it sure was fun when I was nursing my two daughters. I went from an A cup to a C cup, and now I am back down even smaller than before. Honey, I shrunk my breasts! But, thanks to the Wonderbra, I have achieved a balanced shape, filling out my bustline. Clothes look better, which makes me feel better and, after all, feeling good about yourself is what it's all about.

This has inspired me to design and offer a new sports bra. The Denise Austin Up-Lift Bra Top, which is perfect to exercise in, or just to feel comfortable in while wearing your sportswear. It has removable uplift pads for extra lift and shape. So many bra tops tend to press against you and flatten your chest. This gives you uplift and a more defined shape.

Just because I'm flat chested doesn't mean I shy away from low-cut tops. You can create your own cleavage without surgery.

What to avoid:

- **Bodysuits, which tend to flatten the upper body. Avoid anything that presses too tightly against the bodice.**

- **Wrap-top blouses, which tend to make you look concave.**

- **Bandeau styles.**

- **Strapless tops or dresses, unless they have a built-in shelf bra.**

- **Stuffing toilet paper in your bra.**

What to look for:

- **Flattering V-necks.**

- **Tailored, low-cut jackets that nip in the waist.**

- **A Wonderbra!**

SUPER SLIMSUITS

Buying a bathing suit is the most traumatic shopping experience there is.

All those mirrors in such a harshly lit dressing room! Even I hate it, but knowing what works best for your figure before you step into the dressing room is the best way to avoid the bathing-suit blues.

Here are quick and easy solutions to accentuate your best features in a swimsuit and disguise your spot problems.

Tip: Try wearing a pair of two-inch heels while trying on bathing suits. Your legs will automatically look slimmer and longer. Also, move around in the dressing room. Look at every angle. Sit down, and test for comfort as well as fit. Remember: I want you to be able to go swimming in whatever suit you choose and burn those calories!

Do you have full hips?

BEST CHOICE: Look for suits that hit above the crease between hip and thigh. Maillots, or two-piece suits with interesting necklines that draw attention away from your hips to your bustline.

WORST CHOICE: Skirted suits, or the bathing dresses. Low-on-the-leg tank suits. Two-piece suits with hot-pants bottom, or boxer shorts.

Do you have a flat chest?

BEST CHOICE: Suits with wide straps and a high neck, bold patterns, styles with built-in bras and padding. Suits with below-the-bust seams. Attractive, low-back maillots, which emphasize a slender silhouette and draw attention to a well-toned back.

WORST CHOICE: Strapless one-piece styles, and bandeau tops. Shapeless tank suits of flimsy material.

Do you have a long torso?

BEST CHOICE: High-cut legs. Suits that land at the bottom of the hip-bone help elongate the leg. (Women with fuller hips, however, should stick to a cut that's lower.) Low necklines: they create the illusion of a shorter torso.
Bikini bottoms that are high cut on the waist; they shorten the midsection and lengthen the legs.
One-piece suits with patterns across the midsection.

WORST CHOICE: Skimpy string bikinis, dangly details that create more of a vertical illusion.

Do you have a thick waist?

BEST CHOICE: Anything that slims and lengthens the body through waist definition. Look for suits that have details such as a belt or bold stripe across the midsection. Choose high-neck one-piece suits in dark colors for a flattering, slenderizing effect. High-cut legs are flattering on you, and they help create a curvier look at the hip.
Horizontal stripes across the hips can make them look more shapely, and a bright-colored belt helps define the midsection.

WORST CHOICE: Monochromatic suits with no shape or pattern. They will only emphasize your square shape.

ABOUT THE AUTHOR

At 5'4" and 112 pounds, Denise Austin has been dubbed "America's favorite fitness expert." Born on February 13, 1957, Denise grew up in San Pedro, California. She started gymnastics at the age of twelve and earned an athletic scholarship to the University of Arizona, graduating in 1979 with a degree in Exercise Physiology. She began teaching aerobic exercise classes in the Los Angeles area, earning her own local television program two years later. In 1983, Denise married Jeff Austin, a sports attorney and brother of tennis champ Tracy Austin. They moved to Washington, D.C., when Jeff accepted a job with a sports marketing firm.

From 1984–1988, Denise was the resident fitness expert on NBC's *Today* show. She also wrote a column for the *Washington Post* and received a prestigious award from the President's Council on Physical Fitness and Sports.

In 1987 Denise created her ESPN television show, *Getting Fit,* which aired for ten years on ESPN and in eighty-two countries. In January 1997 Denise began her new show, *Denise Austin's Daily Workout* on Lifetime TV. Today she spends four months a year taping her popular program at the most beautiful resorts in the world, traveling with her family as often as possible.

Denise has created twenty-five exercise videos, has her own line of workout equipment, a signature shoe and bodywear by Spalding. She appears monthly on QVC. She can be seen motivating people on talk shows and is often used as a fitness expert for magazine articles. Her sensible, realistic and enthusiastic approach to fitness (she works out only 30 minutes a day) and eating (she never skips a meal) has won fans throughout the United States, from whom she receives over 700 letters a week. Making a difference in the lives of people and her strong belief that she can inspire people to feel better about themselves are what gives Denise the energy to tackle challenges and achieve her success.

A dynamo of energy in a size 5, Denise Austin is a true motivator and has become a veritable fitness empire. But Denise believes her greatest achievement yet is being a mom to her two daughters, Kelly and Katie.

ONCE AGAIN, DENISE AUSTIN DEFINES "SURVIVAL OF THE FITTEST."

"I get so many letters from people saying they just can't find the time to exercise. That's why I created *Hit the Spot*, a series of short, no-nonsense, 30-minute videos that everyone can afford...that every woman can find time to use...and that zero in on the four areas my viewers are concerned about most—their arms, hips, thighs, and butts."

—Denise Austin

It's a fact...

Denise Austin is the most watched and most listened to exercise expert in the world. Her ESPN show, *Getting Fit with Denise Austin*, is seen by over 1 million people a day in the U.S. and countless more millions in 25 countries throughout the world.

To order, call: 1-800-272-4214
PPI Entertainment Group
88 St. Francis Street
Newark, NJ 07105
Copyright 1995 Parade Video/Peter Pan Industries, Inc.

After selling over 5 million videos, Denise Austin hits the spot with exact what her fans wan now—target spo workouts for buns thighs, arms, and abs, all at a very affordable price.

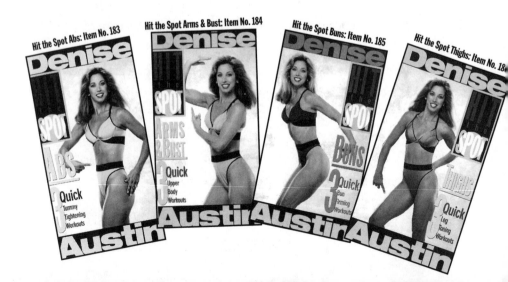

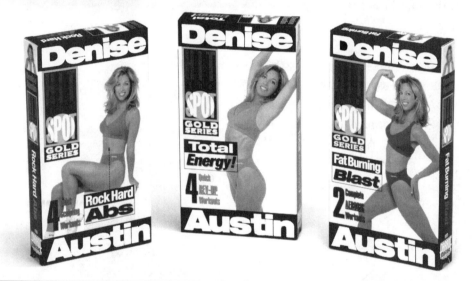

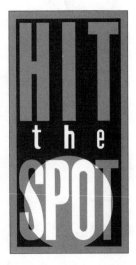